PHARMACISTS TALKING WITH PATIENTS
WITH PATIENTS
A Guide to Patient Counseling

PHARMACISTS TALKING WITH PATIENTS
A Guide to Patient Counseling

Melanie J. Rantucci, BScPharm, MScPharmAd, PhD

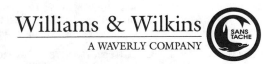

Williams & Wilkins
A WAVERLY COMPANY

BALTIMORE • PHILADELPHIA • LONDON • PARIS • BANGKOK
BUENOS AIRES • HONG KONG • MUNICH • SYDNEY • TOKYO • WROCLAW

1997

ACF - 1683

Editor: Donna Balado
Managing Editor: Victoria Vaughn
Production Coordinator: Felecia R. Weber
Book Project Editor: Susan Rockwell
Cover Designer: Arlene Putterman
Typesetter: Graphic World
Printer: Edwards Brothers
Binder: Edwards Brothers

Accurate indications, adverse reactions and dosage schedules for drugs are provided in this book, but it is possible that they may change. The reader is urged to review the package information data of the manufacturers of the medications mentioned.

Printed in the United States of America.

First Edition,

Library of Congress Cataloging-in-Publication Data

Rantucci, Melanie J.
      Pharmacists talking with patients : a guide to patient counseling
      / Melanie J. Rantucci. -- 1st ed.
          p. cm.
          Includes index.
          ISBN 0-683-07127-0
          1. Pharmacist and patient. 2. Health counseling. I. Title.
          [DNLM: 1. Pharmacists. 2. Counseling--methods. 3. Professional-
          Patient Relations. QV 21 R213p 1997]
      RS56.R36 1997
      362.1'782--dc20
DNLM/DLC
for Library of Congress   96--15264
      CIP

The publishers have made every effort to trace the copyright holders for borrowed material. If they have inadvertently overlooked any, they will be pleased to make the necessary arrangements at the first opportunity.

To purchase additional copies of this book, call our customer service department at **(800) 638-0672** or fax orders to **(800) 447-8438.** For other book services, including chapter reprints and large quantity sales, ask for the Special Sales department.

Canadian customers should call **(800) 268-4178,** or fax **(905) 470-6780.** For all other calls originating outside the United States, please call **(410) 528-4223** or fax us at **(410) 528-8550.**

Visit Williams & Wilkins on the Internet: **http://www.wwilkins.com** or contact our customer service department at **custserv@wwilkins.com.** Williams & Wilkins customer service representatives are available from 8:30 am to 6:00 pm, EST, Monday through Friday, for telephone access.

97 98 99

1 2 3 4 5 6 7 8 9 10

Acknowledgments

I would like to thank Dr. Peggy Piacik, College of Pharmacy, University of Kentucky for making suggestions and providing references to ensure that the content is appropriate for American pharmacists and for suggesting materials to use in Appendix A. In addition, she provided encouragement that indeed this book would be a useful reference for American pharmacists and pharmacy students.

The patient-counseling situations presented at intervals throughout this book were adapted from articles written by this author, printed in the regular pharmacy column "On Counselling" in the Canadian pharmacy journal, *Pharmacy Practice,* published by Thomson Healthcare Communications.

Contents

INTRODUCTION

The topics covered in this book, and their presentation in the context of realistic situations, are intended to help pharmacists and pharmacy students become effective and efficient patient counselors. At the same time, this book will help pharmacists gain more satisfaction from their careers through helping their patients.

Pharmacists and pharmacy students ask many questions about patient counseling. This book is intended to help them find the answers to the these questions.

Why Do Pharmacists Need to Become Involved in Patient Counseling?

With the advent of premanufactured pharmaceuticals, an expanded role for dispensary assistants, and the concept of pharmaceutical care, the technical side of pharmacy has diminished for the community pharmacist, and its more social aspects have become increasingly important. Although pharmacists have always made an effort to know their clientele, and the public have traditionally seen pharmacists as a source of health information, a greater emphasis is now being placed on the patient–pharmacist interaction. In addition, federal legislation and various state regulations now require pharmacists to provide patient counseling to various degrees.

By becoming active in patient counseling, pharmacists can simultaneously derive personal satisfaction and benefit their profession and their business. The first chapter of this book discusses such benefits of patient counseling and illustrates how we as pharmacists can become more successful through effective patient counseling.

What Is Patient Counseling?

The pharmacist is in an ideal position both to ensure that drugs are used in the safest and most effective way possible, and to encourage appropriate self-care. In addition, since people trust pharmacists as educated and approachable health professionals, they often present them with a variety of nonmedication-related questions concerning such issues as birth control or alcohol abuse.

The interaction between pharmacist and patient about such subjects is what patient counseling is all about. Chapter 2 discusses the meaning of the term *patient counseling* and the goals of counseling from the perspective of both the pharmacist and the patient.

How Can We Convert Our Pharmaceutical and Therapeutic Knowledge Into Effective Patient Counseling?

For practical purposes in our day-to-day practices, we need to be able to use our pharmaceutical and therapeutic knowledge to help our patients receive the most benefit from the medications we provide. In order to do this, we must understand our patients and their needs regarding medication use. Chapters 3 and 4 discuss how people feel about being ill and using medication, why they may be noncompliant in their use of medication, and ways in which they may need our help.

What Techniques Are Involved in Patient Counseling?

To become efficient and effective in patient counseling, the pharmacist needs to become adept at using various techniques. Chapter 5 outlines protocols for proceeding with the various types of counseling encounters. To further assist pharmacists in counseling patients, Chapter 6 reviews methods and techniques for providing educational material, and various resources available.

Many of the techniques involved in patient counseling are based on communication theories. The patient–pharmacist interaction should consist of a two-way discussion. Chapter 7 presents selected communication skills necessary for effective patient counseling.

Although patient counseling primarily involves communication between the pharmacist and the patient, contemporary pharmacy practice also involves interacting with other individuals. Chapter 7 therefore includes a discussion about interactions with peers, particularly other health professionals, illustrating how the techniques used in patient counseling can also enhance our relationships within the health-care team.

Each patient and each counseling situation is different. Chapter 8 discusses specific difficulties affecting counseling and counseling for different groups of patients.

Pharmacists also occasionally become aware of nonmedication situations such as unwanted pregnancy, drug and alcohol abuse, and psychological problems, but often feel at a loss as to how to respond to them. Although problems of this nature generally require the input of other providers of care, pharmacists can be of some assistance. This area of social counseling will be discussed in Chapter 8.

How Can I Put Counseling into My Practice?

Although most pharmacists have the desire to counsel patients, they often find the process difficult to implement. Chapter 9 deals with barriers to counseling and ways in which they can be overcome.

The appendices contain additional useful information to help implement patient counseling. Appendix A lists resources available for further study of communication and patient counseling, as well as resources that pharmacists can provide to patients. Since the wording we use to gather information and to express facts and concepts can be critical in patient counseling, Appendix B includes sample dialogues that might be useful as a guideline for the pharmacist and pharmacy student.

Pharmacists must be able to document their actions in patient counseling, such as medication history interviewing and nonprescription drug counseling. In order to be efficient in this pharmacists can use certain forms. Examples of such forms are provided in Appendix C.

How Can I Benefit from a Book About Patient Counseling?

Pharmacists should draw on their own strengths and wealth of experience to interpret the concepts presented in this book in terms of their own needs. Just as each patient and each situation is unique, so too is each pharmacist and each practice setting. In addition, certain jurisdictions require pharmacists to provide various levels of patient counseling. Pharmacists must decide for themselves how patient counseling, as discussed in this book, can fit into their own practices, and what adjustments need to be made to allow for its inclusion. Individual State Board of Pharmacy Regulations must also be reviewed along with the material presented here, and whichever is more stringent should be followed. Pharmacists also need to examine themselves to identify the skills they already have, and the areas in which they must focus their development of new skills.

For pharmacy students, this book will provide an overview of patient counseling. It should be used in adjunct with more comprehensive training in basic communication skills and further discussion of topics in social and administrative pharmacy.

This book is not intended to provide a complete education in patient counseling, simply because patient counseling cannot be learned from reading a book. All pharmacists have the potential to counsel patients—they have the knowledge, the opportunity, and the inherent ability to communicate. The concepts presented will help pharmacists and pharmacy students become aware of their own strengths and identify areas that they need to focus on to become more effective in counseling their patients.

1
PATIENT COUNSELING AS A PHARMACY SERVICE

Pharmacists today are aware that the practice of pharmacy has evolved over the years to include not only preparation and dispensing of medication to patients, but also interaction with patients and other health-care providers throughout the provision of pharmaceutical care. Although pharmacists were originally prevented from discussing therapies with their patients, the American Pharmaceutical Association now includes "initiating pharmacist–patient dialogue" in its professional standards.[1] Patient–pharmacist dialogue is accomplished through patient counseling. Still a pharmacy student may ask "Why should pharmacists spend extra time and effort to counsel? My professors tell me that patient counseling is part of pharmacy practice today, but I wonder if it's really worth the hassle."

Pharmacist A: We should counsel patients because they need it.

Pharmacist B: Pharmacists need to counsel for their own personal legal, professional, and economic reasons.

Pharmacy Student: Which one of you is right?

Both pharmacists and patients benefit from pharmacists' patient-counseling efforts.

Benefits of Patient Counseling to the Patient

In the practice philosophy of pharmaceutical care pharmacists are responsible directly to the patients they serve.[2] The prime motivation for pharmacists to become involved in patient counseling should therefore be benefits to patients through improved quality of life and quality care. The occurrences of so-called "drug misadventures"[3] (adverse effects, side effects, drug interactions, errors in the use of medication) and noncompliance with treatment programs illustrate the need for interventions. In addition, the high costs of health care today call for interventions to minimize waste and to maximize benefits of medical treatments.

As evidence of this need, more than 200 studies and estimates of medication use by nonhospitalized patients suggest that 50% of patients will use their medications incorrectly.[4]

According to a report by the Department of Health and Human Services (HHS) in 1990, 48% of the U.S. population, and 55% of the elderly, fail to comply in some way with their medication regimens.[1] In addition, one study reported that 32% of patients who were instructed by their doctors to have their prescriptions refilled failed to do so.[5] As further evidence of this, it has been calculated that, of the 25,815 prescriptions that could possibly be refilled in the average independent community pharmacy in 1988, only 14,681 were dispensed.[6] In other words, every second or third patient who receives a prescription is likely to use it incorrectly!

Although not all errors are serious enough to impair health, studies again show that 25% of patients will use a medication in a way that does pose a threat to their health.[4] Noncompliance may result in prolonging or increasing the severity of an illness. It may also result in the physician's assuming—on the basis of poor response to the medication—that the illness was misdiagnosed, leading to more tests and possibly additional medication. A recent review of the literature determined that 5.5% of hospital admissions can be attributed to drug therapy noncompliance.[7]

Pharmacists can have a significant impact on these figures through patient counseling. According to the DHHS report "Medication Regimens: Causes of Noncompliance," lack of information about drugs is one of the four most significant "variables that have the most bearing on reasons why the elderly may fail to comply with their medication regimens."[1] Many studies have demonstrated the effectiveness of pharmacist provision of information and compliance reminders. For example, a study in Memphis, Tennessee, found compliance rates of 84.7% for patients receiving a high level of information about an antibiotic drug, compared with 63% for patients receiving less information.[1] Another study improved compliance with cardiac, antihypertensive, and oral hypoglycemic medications by 49% through a prescription-reminder system.[6]

In addition to problems with compliance, patients may suffer adverse drug reactions. Since 1969, approximately 400,000 adverse reactions have been reported to the U.S. Food and Drug Administration, and in 1987, 20% of the cases resulted in either death or hospitalization.[3] Furthermore, occurrences of adverse reactions are substantially underreported; as few as 10% are reported.[2,3] A report by the American Association of Retired Persons indicates that 40% of elderly Americans taking prescription drugs experience adverse effects.[3] Patients may be spared some of these problems if they are made aware of the early signs of adverse drug reactions to report, and if pharmacists inquire about ongoing therapy, allowing early detection and treatment.

In addition to noncompliance and adverse drug reactions, Hepler and Strand list many other drug-related problems: untreated indications, improper drug selection, subtherapeutic dosage, overdosage, drug interactions, and drug use without indication.[2]

These problems may result not only in increased risks for the patient, but also in extra time and expense. In a California study, the cost of hospitalization of elderly patients suffering from adverse drug reactions was found to be $340.1 million.[1] The cost of noncompliance with drug therapy has been estimated as 20 million lost work days and $1.5 billion in lost earnings annually, as well as $8.5 billion in unnecessary hospital expenditures in 1986, approximately 1.7% of all health care expenditures that year.[6,7] Overall, the annual cost of drug-related morbidity in the United States was estimated as early as 1976 to be $7 billion.[8] With costs in health care escalating each year, it is important to patients individually and as tax-payers that pharmacists become involved in patient counseling.

In addition to reducing drug-related morbidity and its subsequent costs to the individual and society, patient counseling may benefit patients in a number of other ways concerning quality of life. Patients may want reassurance that a medication is safe and effective. They may also need additional explanations about their illness that they did not receive from their physician because they were too rushed, too upset, or too embarrassed to ask.

Counseling can further assist patients with self-care. Although many conditions are self-treatable, patients often need help in determining which symptoms are appropriate to self-treat and which need the attention of a physician. Nonprescription-drug misuse has been reported in the literature, with rates varying from 15% to 66% of study groups.[9,10,11] Self-treatment, when appropriate, can reduce the need for and costs of more formal care. As with prescription counseling, pharmacists counseling for non-prescription medications can benefit patients both medically and financially.

Finally, patients may benefit from counseling by pharmacists in non-medication-related situations. There appears to be a gap in the social and health-care system regarding access to treatment. Patients are often unsure where to go for help with a variety of problems ranging from family planning to emotional problems. As available and approachable health professionals, pharmacists can fill this gap and help patients to locate the appropriate social and health-care services. Pharmacists in ambulatory care are often the first contact with the health care system, and as such can coordinate services for the patient and family, as well as provide continuity of care.[12]

Table 1.1 Benefits of Patient Counseling to the Patient

1. *Reduced errors in using medication*

2. *Reduced noncompliance*

3. *Reduced adverse drug reactions*

4. *Reassurance that a medication is safe and effective*

5. *Additional explanations about their illness*

6. *Assistance with self-care*

7. *Referral for assistance with non-drug-related situations (e.g., family*

   planning, emotional problems.)

8. *Reduction in health-care costs to individual, government and society.*

Benefits of Patient Counseling to the Pharmacist

Patient counseling can bring the pharmacist legal, personal, professional and economic benefits, and many new opportunities.

From the legal standpoint, the Omnibus Budget Reconciliation Act of 1990 (OBRA-'90) requires pharmacists to provide patient counseling for Medicaid patients.[13]

Congress outlined the items to be included in patient counseling as a minimum, but it was left up to each state to legislate specific regulations regarding patient counseling.[13] These regulations may change with time, and each pharmacist should consult his or her respective state board of pharmacy to determine the final rules or compliance requirements in any state.

OBRA-'90 requires that an "offer to counsel" must be made, and most states require this to be done by a pharmacist, although some states allow a designate or do not address the question.[14,15] States also vary on whether patients receiving refill prescriptions as well as those receiving new prescriptions need to be counseled and on the use of written information. A few states make the regulation mandatory only for Medicaid patients, but societal and professional pressures require that all patients, not just Medicaid recipients, be counseled. Legal challenges could be made based on the concept of different standards of care being established.[15] Therefore, even in states where counseling is mandated only for Medicaid patients, all patients should be included.

Historically, most courts have held that pharmacists do not have a duty to counsel or warn patients of potential dangers regarding their drug therapy when a prescription is proper on its face and neither the physician nor the drug manufacturer have indicated that warnings need to be given.[15] More recent cases have held that pharmacists have a duty to warn patients in certain situations, and the new OBRA-'90 regulations will probably confirm this.[15] The number of criminal prosecutions and disciplinary actions has increased in recent years, and it is anticipated that future legal cases will focus not only on whether regulations were complied with, but also on the quality (i.e. accuracy and completeness) of the pharmacist's performance of the OBRA-'90 mandates.[16] Although some pharmacists may feel concern over these legal implications of patient counseling, complying with state requirements can be expected to reduce the risk of being sued about consulting and to put pharmacists in a better position to defend themselves should a patient make a claim, particularly if actions involving patient counseling are documented.[16]

Pharmacists' involvement in patient counseling can also benefit pharmacists professionally. The technical and mechanical functions of pharmacists may easily be replaced in the future. We are seeing many new developments: new drug-delivery systems such as implants; the use of computers, automated prescription vial fillers, and other potential types of automation such as automated teller machines; and new roles for pharmacy technicians.[16] In addition, nurses have already established roles in providing pharmacy services and in counseling patients.[16] Unless pharmacists become involved in all aspects of pharmaceutical care, including patient counseling, they in effect perform the role of technicians, thereby diminishing their professional status.[17]

At the same time, pharmacists are striving to be recognized by patients and other health professionals as important players in the health-care team, that is, the team's experts in the field of drugs. Standards of practice for the profession of pharmacy by the American Pharmaceutical Association and other pharmacy organizations, as well as guidelines for patient counseling by these organizations, promote the role of pharmacists in patient counseling.

In addition, the pharmaceutical care model has become the model for professional practice. To provide complete pharmaceutical care, the pharmacist must carry out each of the nine steps of the pharmaceutical care process as described by Strand and colleagues.[17] During this process the pharmacist must consult with the patient to develop a working relationship; to gather the necessary facts; and to determine the patient's needs and wishes. The pharmacist must inform the patient of the problems identified and work with the patient in identifying solutions, options, and desired outcomes and in developing an individual plan. Through regular discussions with the patient, the pharmacist can ensure that the patient carries out the plan and that the plan is successful from both the pharmacist's and patient's points of view.[17]

Apart from legal and professional inducements to counsel patients, pharmacists have a personal stake in patient-counseling involvement. A diminishing professional status affects pharmacists' self-worth and job satisfaction, which have been found to be related to clinical and professional aspects of the job.[18] In general, pharmacists report that counseling and patient education are the greatest sources of job satisfaction, and that they want to spend more time advising and counseling.[18,19] Patient counseling offers pharmacists a chance to demonstrate professional capabilities and to use the knowledge that they have gained through many years of study. Whereas dispensing tasks alone can be repetitive and unfulfilling, personal interaction can add variety and interest to the pharmacist's job. In addition, there is the personal satisfaction of helping another person, particularly in helping that person to regain or maintain health.

An additional personal benefit for pharmacists' involvement in patient counseling involves job stress. A pharmacist's job can be very stressful at times, primarily as a result of dealing with clients who are often ill and under stress themselves.[20] Through discussion with the patient during counseling, the pharmacist can come to understand the patient's position and gain his or her cooperation, ultimately reducing the level of stress of both patient and pharmacist.[20] The discrepancy between practice expectations and reality is often upsetting to pharmacists, who feel frustrated at not fully using their knowledge. Involvement in patient counseling presents the opportunity for pharmacists to make more comprehensive use of their knowledge.[16]

From the economic and business points of view, pharmacists are realizing that patient counseling, in an environment of tough competition, can be seen as an extra service with the potential to entice customers. It has been observed that "because pharmaceutical products are virtually identical, the only manner in which pharmacies can differentiate themselves is by the services they provide."[21] Indeed, there is ample evidence that patient counseling is a service that the public wants. Many studies have investigated consumers' needs and demands for pharmaceutical services, specifically: both verbal and written information, information on warnings and side effects, explanation of directions, storage directions, poison information, refill status, and brand versus generic information.[21,22]

The advent of preferred provider organizations and the growing number of prescriptions dispensed through mail-order and managed-care pharmacies, serves to emphasize the economic need for pharmacists to enhance the value of personal contact with patients through patient counseling.[16]

In addition, many studies have illustrated that consumers are willing to pay for patient counseling services. A review of these studies indicates that between 26% and 55% of consumers say they would pay from $1 to $5 per session for counseling services when the information presented is tailored to the individual needs of the patient and is provided in a private or semiprivate setting.[22] Recently, pharmaceutical and insurance companies have begun to reimburse pharmacists for patient counseling in specific instances, such as diabetic counseling.[23]

Patient counseling has also been shown to help pharmacists reduce the amount of revenue lost as a result of unfilled or un-refilled prescriptions. Unfilled and un-refilled prescriptions represent a loss of approximately 100 million prescriptions annually.[5] A recent survey of consumers found that 8.7% of the respondents do not fill their initial prescriptions, with a potential value of $2.8 billion or $1000 per week for the average pharmacy.[24] In the average pharmacy, 11,134 prescriptions that are eligible for renewal each year are not refilled, and a 50% increase in refill compliance by verbal reinforcement and reminders could increase net profit by $26,805 (based on average prescription price of $16.60, and expenses of 13% of sales).[6]

It is evident from this discussion that there is more than enough motivation for pharmacists and pharmacy owners to promote and become involved in patient counseling.

Table 1.2   Benefits of Patient Counseling to the Pharmacist

1. *Legal protection, since pharmacists may be held accountable for injury resulting from insufficient information provided to the patient*

2. *Maintenance of professional status as part of the health care team*

3. *Increased job satisfaction*

4. *Reduced job stress*

5. *An added service to attract customers and aid in market competition*

6. *Increased revenue through payment for counseling services and reduced loss resulting from unfilled or un-refilled prescriptions*

References

1. Kessler D. A challenge for American pharmacists. Am Pharm. 1992; NS32(1):33-36.
2. Hepler C, Strand L. Opportunities and responsibilities in pharmaceutical care. Am J Hosp Pharm. 1990;47(3):533-554.
3. Manasse Jr H. Medication use in an imperfect world: Drug misadventuring as an issue of public policy, part 1. Am J Hosp Pharm 1989;46(5):929-943.
4. Sackett D, Snow J. The magnitude of compliance and noncompliance. In: Compliance in health care. Haynes R, Taylor D, Sackett D, eds. Baltimore: Johns Hopkins University Press. 1979:11-22.
5. Schering Laboratories. The forgetful patient: The high cost of improper patient compliance. Schering Report no. 9, Kenilworth, NJ: Schering Laboratories. 1987.
6. Jackson R, Huffman Jr D. Patient compliance: The financial impact on your practice. NARD J. 1990;112(7):67-71.
7. Sullivan SD, Kreling DH, Hazlet TK. Noncompliance with medication regimens and subsequent hospitalization: A literature analysis and cost of hospitalization estimate. J Res Pharm Econ. 1990;2(2):19-34.
8. McKenney TJ, Harrison WR. Drug-related hospital admissions. Am J Hosp Pharm. 1976;33(8):792-795.
9. Wilkinson I, Darby D, Mant A. Self-care and self-medication: An evaluation of individuals' health care decisions. Med Care. 1987;25(10): 965-978.
10. Salerno E, Ries D, San J, et al. Self-medication behaviors. Fla J Hosp Pharm. 1985;5(7):13-28.
11. Shimp L, Ascione F, Glazer H et al. Potential medication-related problems in non-institutionalized elderly. DICP. 1985;19(10):766-772.
12. Plein J. Pharmacy's paradigm: Welcoming the challenges and realizing the opportunities. Am J Pharm Ed. 1992;56(4):283-287.
13. Martin S. What you need to know about OBRA-'90. Am Pharm. 1993;NS33(1):26-28.
14. Anon. APhA Surveys states on counseling laws. Am Pharm. 1993;NS33(3):23-24.
15. Ginsberg D, Bair T. States put Medicaid law into practice. Drug Topics. 1993;137(1):18-20,23.
16. Portner T, Fitzgerald Jr WJ. OBRA-'90:Turning a challenge into an opportunity. Am Pharm. 1993;NS33(3):67-75.
17. Strand LM, Cipolle RJ, Morley PC. Pharmaceutical care: An introduction. Current concepts, 1992. Kalamazoo, MI: The UpJohn Co., 1992:15.
18. Anderson-Harper H, Berger B, Noel R. Pharmacists' predisposition to communicate, desire to counsel and job satisfaction. Am J Pharm Ed. 1992;56(4)252-258.
19. Chi J. Inside today's pharmacist 1992. Part 1: Career and work place. Drug Topics. 1992;136(6):47,51-52,57.

20. Rybka-Miki C. Reducing stress in pharmacy practice. On Continuing Practice. 1989;16(2):31-34.
21. Malone D, Rasciti K, Gagnon JP. Consumers' evaluation of value-added pharmacy services. Am Pharm. 1993;NS33(3):48-56.
22. Carroll N. Consumer demand for patient oriented services in community pharmacies: A review and comment. J Soc Admin Pharm 1985:3(2):64-69.
23. Anon. Pharmacist's Letter. 1992;8(9):49.
24. Anon. Schering Report XIV, Kentucky Pharm. 1992;June; 176-179.

2
DEFINING PATIENT COUNSELING

The Meaning of Counseling

Pharmacy Student: What is patient counseling, anyway?

Pharmacist A: Patient counseling is giving advice to patients.

Pharmacist B: Patient counseling is patient education.

Pharmacist C: Patient counseling is truly "counseling" in the same way that professional counselors and therapists use psychotherapy techniques to help their clients deal with problems.

Pharmacy Student: Which of you is right?

When pharmacists talk about patient counseling, they are often referring to a variety of activities. Each pharmacist may have a different idea of what patient counseling involves. To some, it is the education of the patient about his or her medication; to others, patient counseling involves a broader range of activities.

The words *counseling, consulting*, and *patient education* are often used interchangeably by pharmacists, but they actually connote different activities and approaches. The word *counsel* is defined in the dictionary as giving advice, but it also implies mutual discussion and an exchange of opinions.[1,2] To *consult* means to seek advice, and suggests almost exclusively receiving advice rather than exchanging information. Education involves a slightly different sphere of interaction: it is defined in the dictionary as "instruction and development to impart skills and knowledge."[1,2]

The theories underpinning the professional fields of counseling and education offer more comprehensive explanations of these terms. In counseling theory, for example, counseling is considered similar, in many ways, to psychotherapy.[3] Counseling and psychotherapy involve the same activities, but place emphasis on different areas. Both involve listening, questioning, evaluating, interpreting, supporting, explaining, informing, advising, and ordering. However, the main emphasis in psychotherapy is on listening, whereas counseling puts the emphasis equally on listening and informing.[3]

In educational theory, education connotes much more than simply imparting knowledge. It may be defined as "progressive changes of a person affecting knowledge, attitudes, and behavior as a result of instruction and study."[4] Education involves processes through which people develop their abilities, and enrich their knowledge and which help to bring about changes in their attitudes or behavior.[5]

From this semantic discussion, it may be seen that the activity that pharmacists refer to as "patient counseling" involves counseling in the psychological sense, as well as activities that aim to educate patients. It encompasses theories of counseling and education in varying degrees, depending on the situation and the needs of the patient.

Understanding the Counseling Perspective

Since a large component of patient counseling is counseling in the psychological sense, it is useful to understand some of the roots of counseling theory.

Behavioral Aspects of Pharmacy Counseling

An important basis of counseling theory is the theory of behavior drawn from the work of B.F. Skinner, who suggested that behavior that is reinforced (rewarded) is repeated and, conversely, behavior that is not reinforced or that is actually punished is not repeated.[6]

A broader approach is cognitive behavior modification.[6] It assumes that it is not the experience alone that is the cause of behavior, it is the individual's underlying cognition of the experience (conceptions, ideas, meanings, beliefs, thoughts, inferences, expectations, predictions, or attributions).[7] These cognitions vary from individual to individual and are acquired throughout the course of life through experiences.[7]

Through counseling, by persuasion and argument, the individual's false assumptions, irrational conclusions, and misconceptions will be changed so that he or she thinks, feels, and behaves on a more rational basis.[7]

Thus, when explaining to the patient the reasons behind medication instructions and the ways in which the medication will treat the condition, the pharmacist attempts to change the patient's thoughts about the usefulness of the medication and the importance of compliance. This change in the patient's thoughts is expected to result in a behavioral change with regard to compliance.

Behavior therapy is the source of some of the patient education methods that will be described in Chapters 4 and 6, such as self-monitoring, demonstration (modelling), and practice (behavior rehearsal).

Theories of Health Behavior

Theories of health behavior are also important to the development of communication skills used in patient counseling. There have been many attempts to analyze why patients behave the way they do when they are ill and need to take medication. Theories of health behavior suggest that patients' perceptions about the severity and possible outcome of their condition, the effectiveness and benefits of medication use, and various triggers to taking medication may be critical elements in patient medication use. This will be discussed further in Chapter 3.

These theories indicate that patient counseling involves not only an exchange of information, but should also involve an attempt to change the patient's health beliefs.

Humanist Approaches to Counseling

The humanist school of psychology considers peoples' thoughts and feelings in addition to behaviors.[8] When pharmacists counsel patients they should acknowledge that patients are not only behaving (acting) due to external controls of stimulus and reward, but that they are also thinking and feeling.

When a patient is noncompliant, not only is he acting by not taking his medication, but he is doing so because of thoughts and feelings about his illness and medication use. As a result, pharmacists' counseling should take the patient's feelings and thoughts into consideration.

The person-centered approach to counseling, developed by Carl Rogers, is part of humanistic psychology and is one of the greatest influences on the field of counseling.[7] This approach to counseling is based on the idea that people will naturally grow and develop their capacities (self-actualization). A person is able to solve his or her own problems in a relationship with a helping person that is nonjudgmental and where the person feels cared for, genuinely and unconditionally.[8]

From this perspective, the pharmacist helps patients get the most benefit from their therapy by helping them to feel capable of controlling their own medication use, in other words, by helping them to identify and solve their own problems in this area.

A key element of this helping approach is the pharmacist's genuine feelings of warmth and concern for patients and his or her trust in their abilities to solve their own problems.[8] This is exemplified in part by the pharmacist taking the necessary time to spend with each patient, and by the pharmacist's helping attitude during the interaction.

An Eclectic Counseling Theory

The process of helping described by Egan involves three stages: 1) clarifying the problem (to explore the individual's viewpoint of the problem); 2) setting goals (achieving an overview of the individual's problems and set goals to overcome them; and 3) facilitating action (to help the person plan ways of achieving the goals set, to carry out the goals and to evaluate the outcomes).[7]

This helping process will be further elaborated later in this chapter.

Counseling Goals

"Counseling," as defined, then is essentially a helping process.[9] In order to do this, the pharmacist must establish a relationship with the patient and develop trust.[10] The pharmacist also needs to demonstrate concern and care for the patient in order for him to know that the information the pharmacist is providing and the questions the pharmacist is asking are in the patient's interest.[10]

What is it that the patient needs help with? The essence of all counseling is to help a person cope effectively with an important problem or concern.[9] In the case of patient medication counseling, that problem involves the individual's health and the need to fit medication use into his or her daily life. For example, a patient may need help in planning how he can take an antibiotic every 6 hours, when he is at work part of the day and asleep at night.

Patient counseling might also involve helping the patient to cope with illness and with the changes it is likely to bring about in his or her lifestyle. For example, patients with illnesses such as diabetes and high blood pressure may require help in coping with changes in diet as well as changes in work habits and recreational activities.

In addition to dealing with immediate problems, counseling involves interventions to prevent the occurrence of later problems and to develop the individual's capacity to deal with such problems if they should arise.[11] In the case of patient medication counseling, problems can be anticipated and then prevented or at least minimized through discussion with the patient. Future problems might involve the patient's ability and intention to comply with the medication directions. For example, a patient going to a party might decide to skip one of his prescribed high blood pressure pills so that he can enjoy a potentially interacting alcoholic beverage at the party. If such situations have been anticipated and discussed with the pharmacist, then the patient can make better decisions when the time comes. The pharmacist could point out the risks of missing a dose of the medication and suggest alternatives to the patient such as restricting himself to nonalcoholic beverages, such as mineral water with lemon, while taking the medication.

Other future problems might involve the development of side effects or adverse effects. The occurrence of side effects such as constipation or discolored urine may alarm or disturb a patient sufficiently to cause him to discontinue the medication. If the patient is forewarned, however, he will recognize the symptom as a side effect and know how to handle it (e.g., use a stool softener for constipation), while continuing on the medication.

Similarly, if a patient is told about the signs of possible adverse effects, then such effects can be detected at an early stage, and the physician can be notified before more serious effects set in. In addition, patients who fear possible adverse effects will be reassured by knowing how rarely they occur and by understanding how they can be detected at an early stage, or even modified. The unknown is often more frightening than the known. Knowing what to expect and what action to take allows the patient to exert some control over unavoidable events.

In the case of repeat medications, the goal of counseling is to detect any of the above problems and ensure that things are proceeding well.

Once present and future problems with medication use have been detected, the goal of counseling is to develop the patient's capacity to deal with such problems. Although some problems will involve the intervention of the physician and perhaps other health professionals (e.g., community visiting nurse), the patient is still an integral part of the problem solution.

Through counseling, the pharmacist can explore the patient's present and future needs. The pharmacist must discover what the patient needs to know; what skills he or she needs to develop; and what problems need to be dealt with. In addition, the pharmacist must determine which behaviors and attitudes need to be modified.

The techniques involved in counseling the patient in order to attain these goals will be discussed in Chapters 5, 6, 7 and 8.

Table 2.1   Counseling Goals

1. To establish a relationship with the patient and to develop trust

2. To demonstrate concern and care for the patient

3. To help the patient manage and adapt to his or her medication

4. To help the patient manage and adapt to his or her illness

5. To prevent or minimize problems associated with side effects, adverse effects, or present and future noncompliance

6. To develop the patient's capacity to deal with such problems

Educational Goals

To attain the counseling goals of helping the patient in various ways, the pharmacist must also take steps to enhance patients' skills and knowledge about their illnesses and their medications in order to bring about necessary changes in related attitudes and behaviors. This is the essence of the "educational" goals of patient counseling.

Pharmacists often think of education as providing verbal or written information. Simply providing information, however, does not guarantee that patients' skills and knowledge will improve, or that their behavior and attitudes will be affected.

The pharmacist's educational goal will be to provide information that meets the specific needs of each patient. Through discussion with a patient, the pharmacist must first determine how much the patient already knows about the medication in question, and whether he or she holds any misconceptions about the medication or the illness it is meant to treat. For example, a patient may believe that his high blood pressure is the result of bad nerves; that "hypertensive" medication is meant to relieve "tension"; and that the medication is needed only when he is feeling "hyper." On discovering that the patient holds such views, the pharmacist will know that he must convey clear information about the meaning of high blood pressure; the purpose of the medication; and the importance of taking the medication regularly.

The educational goals of patient counseling also involve investing patients with the skills and techniques they need to optimize their prescribed therapy. For example, a patient may need instruction in the proper use of an inhaler or assistance in devising a method for remembering and following a complicated dosage schedule.

Finally, the pharmacist must provide information and instruction in a way that makes them effective for *this* particular patient in *this* particular situation. For example, the information and instructional methods required by a young patient receiving an inhaler for the first time will be quite different from those needed by an elderly patient receiving a new prescription for diabetes treatment in addition to several repeat prescriptions treating arthritis and congestive heart failure. The approach taken in the educational process is an important aspect of dealing with the individual needs of the particular patient and the particular situation.

Table 2.2   Educational Goals

1. *To provide information appropriate to the particular individual and the particular problem*

2. *To provide skills and methods that the patient can use to optimize the usage and effects of the medication*

3. *To present information and instruction using educational methods that are appropriate to the particular individual and the particular situation*

Patient Counseling as an Integral Component of Pharmaceutical Care

Since the introduction of the concept of pharmaceutical care, the role of patient counseling in the model of pharmacy practice has often been relegated to a box off in the corner involving the provision of patient information. From the discussion, it is evident that patient counseling is a large component of pharmaceutical care, and is necessary throughout the process. The American Society of Health System Pharmacists' guidelines on pharmacist-conducted patient counseling state that "pharmacist-conducted patient counseling is a component of pharmaceutical care and should be aimed at improving therapeutic outcomes by maximizing proper use of medications."[12]

Throughout the Pharmaceutical Care Process described by Strand et al., each step requires patient–pharmacist interaction: establishing the pharmacist–patient relationship; collecting and interpreting patient information; listing and ranking drug-related problems; determining desired pharmacotherapeutic goals; determining feasible alternatives; selecting and individualizing the most appropriate treatment regimen; designing a drug-monitoring plan; implementing the decisions about drug use; designing a monitoring plan to achieve desired therapeutic goals and following-up to determine the success of treatment.[13] In fact, this seems to mirror the three stages of the helping process as outlined by Egan described earlier: problem clarification, setting goals, and facilitating action.

Particularly in the community pharmacy setting, the *patient* is the main source of information. The *patient* must contribute to identifying problems and should play a role in deciding desired goals, alternatives, and treatment regimens. The *patient* must be consulted with, to implement the plan and to monitor its outcomes.

Strand et al. refer to pharmaceutical care as an "integrated patient-specific model of pharmacy practice," and assert that, to deliver pharmaceutical care "the pharmacist must see the patient, explain the proposed relationship, discuss the various choices, obtain information, and seek cooperation, trust, and permission."[13,14] Indeed, patient counseling is interwoven throughout the pharmaceutical care model and is an integral part of it.

The Pharmacist's Approach to Patient Counseling

Now that the goals of patient counseling have been discussed, the approach that pharmacists need to take to attain these goals should be considered. As discussed above, the goals involve helping and educating the patient; it follows, then, that the pharmacist must approach the patient-counseling encounter as a helper and an educator.

The Helping Approach

The "helper" role for pharmacists has been clearly identified in the provisional draft mission statement for pharmacy practice developed by the Joint Commission on Pharmacy Practice: "The mission of pharmacy practice is to help people make the best use of medications."[15]

Pharmacists have traditionally been involved in the preparation and dispensing of medication, at the direction of the physician. As such, they have been strongly allied with the medical profession and, hence, with the view that the health professional should be in control of the patient. But, with the shift in the model of pharmacy from a focus on the medication to a focus on the patient, there is a need for a shift in the pharmacist's approach as well. This shift can be described as moving from the health professional-centered "medical model" approach to the patient-centered "helping model" approach.

The medical model and the helping model contrast with respect to the relationship between the health professional and the patient, which differs in the two models in a number of areas: the role of each party in the relationship; the basis for trust; the approach to problem solving; and the allowance for the solving of future problems.[16]

In the medical model, the health professional is active and the patient is passive; in the helping model, both patient and health professional are active. In the medical model, the basis for trust is the presumed expertise and authority of the health professional, to which the patient automatically responds. In the helping model, trust is not automatic, but grows slowly, based on the personal relationship – trust develops mutually between the professional and the patient.

Although in both models a need to solve a problem is the reason for the relationship, their approaches to problem-solving are considerably different. In the medical model, the health professional identifies the problem, analyzes information, arrives at a diagnosis, and gives direction to work on the solution. The patient is responsible only for answering questions and following directions. In the helping model, the professional assists the patient in exploring the problem and possible solutions. The patient is responsible for drawing conclusions, making decisions, and selecting a solution he or she can follow.

In the medical model, the patient becomes dependent on the professional. As a result, the patient must return to the health professional to deal with future problems in the previously learned way and to seek help if necessary. In the helping model, the patient develops self-confidence to manage his or her own problems.

The relationship between the health professional and the patient in the medical model is more akin to a parent–child relationship than to the equal, adult relationship that characterizes the helping model.

The comparison described is very black and white, and is probably an oversimplification of what is indeed a complicated process.[16] In reality, a range of approaches exists, on a continuum from the health professional-centered medical-model approach to the patient-centered helping model approach. Pharmacists must decide for themselves where on the continuum they feel most comfortable in their relationship with the patient, and also where the patient may feel most comfortable. To attain the counseling goals most effectively, however, the pharmacist must lean more heavily toward the helping-model approach.

Table 2.3   The Helping Approach: Relationship between Health Professional and Patient

Medical Model	Helping Model
Patient is passive	*Patient is actively involved*
Basis for trust is expertise and authority of health professional	*Trust is based on personal relationship developed over time*
Health professional identifies problems and determines solutions	*Health professional assists patient in exploring problem and possible solutions*
Patient is dependent on health professional	*Patient develops self-confidence to manage problems*
Parent–child relationship	*Equal relationship*

Adapted from Anderson TP. An Alternative Frame of Reference for Rehabilitation: The Helping Process versus the Medical Model. In: Marinelli R, Dell Orto A., eds. The Psychological and Social Impact of Physical Disability. New York: Springer, 1977: 18-20.

The Educational Approach

The approach taken to the educational process is critical to the pharmacist's success in achieving the educational goals of patient counseling. In the majority of cases, patient counseling involves dealing with adults. When pharmacists approach the educational aspects of patient counseling, however, they often become "teachers," adapting a style that they recall from their childhood.

Knowles explains that most of what we know today about the learning process derives from studies of learning in children under conditions of compulsory attendance.[5] The theories and assumptions that guided such studies were termed "pedagogy," from the Greek stem *pais* meaning child, and *agogos* meaning leader. Knowles further explains that, somewhere in history, the "child" part of the definition got lost, so that even the dictionary defines "pedagogy" simply as the art and science of teaching. The result, Knowles suggests, is that most teachers of adults only know how to teach adults as if they were children.[5]

While Knowles does not suggest that there is a fundamental difference between the way adults and the way children learn, he does point out that differences exist in the conditions surrounding adult and child learning and that certain changes occur in the learning process with the student's maturity—hence, the emergence of the term "andragogy," the art and science of helping adults learn.[17]

There are four basic concepts around which differences between andragogy and pedagogy can be illuminated: 1) self-concept; 2) experience; 3) readiness to learn; and 4) time perspective and orientation to learning.[17]

Self-Concept

As children move toward adulthood, their self-concept changes from one of dependency to one of autonomy. They become increasingly aware of their capacity to make decisions for themselves. In pedagogy, the relationship between teacher and learner is a directing one, in which the learner is dependent and the teacher dominant. Because of this, adults tend to resent being treated as though they were children and perceive this as being treated with a lack of respect, being talked down to, or being judged.[17] As a result, patients instructed from a pedagogical approach may not follow medication directions and may not admit to noncompliance or concerns about their conditions since they may fear being ridiculed or scolded.

In andragogy, the relationship between teacher and learner becomes a helping relationship, characterized by reciprocity in the teaching–learning transaction.[17] In educating adult patients, the pharmacist must join with them to help solve problems relating to their illness and medication use.

Experience

Adults accumulate a vast range of experience over the course of their lifetime, which contributes to the way they view and interpret new experiences, and the way they approach the need for new information.[17]

In relation to illness and medication, patients may have certain beliefs arising out of previous experiences of their own or out of those of others that they have heard about. For example, a patient may have experienced an unpleasant side effect from a medication taken in the past, and therefore, may be reluctant to use medication, even when it is prescribed for the treatment of a life-threatening condition.

In pedagogy, at least in the past, the experience of children was not considered, since it was not expected to be significant. Therefore, educational methods traditionally involved "one-way communication" techniques, such as lectures, readings, and audiovisual presentations. In andragogy, the experience of adults is drawn upon as a resource in learning. Adult learners use their experiences to facilitate the learning process for themselves and others. Two-way communication techniques, such as group discussions, simulation, role playing, and skill-practice sessions, are likely to be more effective.[17]

Pharmacists are therefore best advised to approach counseling with a variety of techniques, rather than simply presenting a lecture about medications. Such techniques will be discussed in Chapters 5 and 6.

Readiness to Learn

In the education of children, the main task lies in sequencing and interrelating subjects and in developing competency in basic skills such as reading, writing, and arithmetic. Adult educational tasks are more closely related to social roles such as working, raising a family, and enjoying recreational activities. The subjects that adults need to learn are usually of immediate concern and importance in their daily lives.[17] For example, a patient may need to learn how to use an inhaler or how to cope with an illness while continuing to work and participate in other social functions.

In pedagogy, teachers decide what will be learned and how and when the learning will take place. In andragogy, adults make themselves available for learning because of their perception of a particular need in a particular area (e.g., in the context of health, the need for assistance with breathing). Adults will choose what they need to know (e.g., how to use an inhaler) and when they want to learn about it (when they pick up the prescription or later, when they have time to talk). Patients must perceive the need for the medication and for proper instruction in its use before they will be prepared to learn about, for example, inhaler use, and make themselves available for the necessary instruction. Rather than forging ahead with instructions, then, the pharmacist must act as a resource person to help patients discover their own learning needs.

Time Perspective and Orientation to Learning

In pedagogy, children acquire information in preparation for the future. Learning is subject-centered, and the teacher serves as a source of knowledge. The andragogical approach to education, on the other hand, is problem-centered: it involves identifying the problem and solving it in the present.[17]

It is up to the pharmacist to discover, from the patient, the kind of information that will be useful for solving that patient's specific problems. Through discussion with the patient, the pharmacist can avoid providing extraneous information – the kind that does not apply to the particular patient or the particular situation. Instructing a patient to avoid operating hazardous machinery while using a medication, for example, is a useless exercise for both the pharmacist and patient if that patient is an 80-year-old woman who neither drives nor works in a factory. The pharmacist must first learn from patients the information that they need to solve their own individual problems, then tailor the counseling to the particular patient. Aspects of "tailoring" in patient counseling will be discussed in Chapter 8.

Table 2.4 The Educational Approach: Conditions and Process of Learning

Pedagogy	Andragogy
Learner is dependent; teacher is dominant	*Helping relationship, with reciprocity in the teaching–learning transaction*
Experience is not considered	*Experience is drawn upon as a resource in learning*
Educational methods involve one-way communication techniques such as lectures, readings, and audiovisual presentations	*Two-way communication techniques such as group techniques, discussions, simulation, role-playing, and skill-practice sessions, are more effective*
Sequencing and interrelating subjects and skill-building activities are used to develop competency in basic skills for the future	*Educational tasks are more closely related to social roles and involve subjects of immediate concern and importance in the individual's daily life*
The teacher decides what will be learned and how and when the learning will take place	*Adults choose what they want to learn, and when*
Learning is subject-centered, and the teacher serves as a source of knowledge	*Learning is problem-centered, and involves identifying and solving the problem in the present*

Adapted from Knowles MS. What is andragogy. In: The Modern Practice of Adult Education. Englewood Cliffs, NJ: Prentice Hall Regents, 1970; 40-62.

Summary

From this discussion, perhaps an overall definition of patient medication counseling may be stated: *Talking with patients about the medications they are intended to take so that they will get the most benefit from the medications.*

This chapter has emphasized that the patient is at the center of the patient counseling approach. Therefore, it is important for the pharmacist to try to understand patients' perspectives in relation to illness and medication use. This will be discussed in the following two chapters.

References

1. Morehead A, Morehead L eds. The New American Webster Dictionary. New American Library Times Mirror. 1972.
2. Funk CE. New Practical Standard Dictionary. New York: Funk and Wagnalls. 1950.
3. Corsini RJ. Introduction. In: Current Psychotherapies. 3d ed. Itasca, IL: FE Peacock Publishers, Inc. 1984:1-13.
4. Lively BT. The community pharmacist and health education. Contemporary Pharmacy Practice. 1982;5:14-20.
5. Knowles MS. What is andragogy. In: The Modern Practice of Adult Education. Englewood Cliffs, NJ. Prentice Hall Regents. 1970:40-62.
6. Wilson G. Behavior therapy. In: Current Psychotherapies. 3rd ed. Corsini R and contributors. Itasca, IL: FE Peacock Publishers, Inc.1984:239-278.
7. Davis H, Fallowfield L. Counseling Theory. In: Counseling and Communication in Health Care. Davis H, Fallowfield L, eds. Chichester, England: John Wiley & Sons. 1991:23-58.
8. Meach B, Rogers C. Person-centered therapy. In: Current Psychotherapies. 3rd ed. Corsini R and contributors. Itasca, IL: FE Peacock Publishers, Inc. 1984:142-195.
9. Eisenberg S, Delaney DJ. The Counseling Process. 2nd ed. Chicago: Rand & McNally. 1977:12-31.
10. Leibowitz K. Improving your patient counseling skills. Am Pharm. 1993:33;465-69.
11. Krumboltz JD, Thoresen CE. Counseling methods. Holt Rinehart and Winston, New York. 1976:1-25.
12. Anon. ASHP guidelines on pharmacy-conducted patient counseling. Am J Hosp Pharm. 1993:50(3);505-506.
13. Strand LM, Cipolle RJ, Morley PC. Pharmaceutical care: an introduction. Current concepts, 1992. Kalamazoo, MI: The UpJohn Co. 1992:15.
14. Strand L, Guerrero R, Nickman N, Morley P. Integrated patient-specific model of pharmacy practice. Am J Hosp Pharm.1990:47(3):550-554.
15. Anon. JCCP provisional draft mission statement for pharmacy practice. NARD Newsletter. Oct. 1, 1991:4.
16. Anderson TP. An alternative frame of reference for rehabilitation: The helping process versus the medical model. In: The Psychological and Social Impact of Physical Disabilities. Marinelli R, Dell Orto AE, eds. New York: Springer. 1977:18-20.
17. Ingalls JD. A Trainer's Guide to Andragogy.Waltham, MA: Data Education, Inc. 1976.

3
UNDERSTANDING PATIENTS' NEEDS, WISHES, AND PREFERENCES

From the preceding discussion about the goals of counseling, it follows that, in each counseling situation, the pharmacist needs to determine the particular needs, wishes and preferences of each individual patient concerning his own health. The specific details of what needs to be done to accomplish those goals for each individual patient need to be determined. Consider the following two patients:

Mrs. Jones is receiving a prescription for high blood pressure and says to the pharmacist, "I know Dr. Harris told me I need this, but I feel fine. My mother and father both lived into their 90s and never needed pills. Maybe I don't really need them."

The next patient, Mr. Hoffman receives a prescription for the same medication as Mrs. Jones. He comments to the pharmacist, "I know my blood pressure is pretty high, and I should be taking these pills regularly, but I have a busy schedule and I find it difficult remembering to take them."

These two patients have different counseling needs. Mrs. Jones needs help in understanding her illness and the necessity to take medication daily, whereas Mr. Hoffman needs help in remembering and scheduling his medication.

Decisions about the patient's needs, preferences, and wishes must be made fairly quickly, sometimes without the aid of complete background information. The specific goals of the counseling can be determined in part through discussion with the patient—by means of open questions and probing. These techniques will be discussed further in Chapter 7.

The pharmacist must also gain a sense of what a patient's feelings and concerns are in order to establish a relationship with the patient, to help direct the discussion, and to decide on an approach to the patient's situation. Pharmacists who have a general understanding of how people feel about being ill and about using medication will have a better idea of how to proceed with the individual counseling session.

Illness versus Sickness: The Patient's Perspective

The World Health Organization defines health as "a state of complete physical, mental, and social well being, and not just the absence of disease and infirmity."[1] Conversely, then, illness can be seen as more than just the presence of disease. The terms "illness" and "sickness" are used interchangeably by most people, but to analysts of health and illness issues, they suggest different perspectives.[2] "Sickness" refers to the limited scientific concept of a diagnosed medical condition, whereas "illness" refers to an individual's perception of any condition that causes that individual to be concerned and seek help. The study of illness behavior, or health-related behavior, considers issues surrounding the individual's perceptions of symptoms.[2]

Symptoms are perceived, evaluated, and acted on (or not acted on) differently by different people and in different social situations.[2] Individuals may differ in their attentiveness to pain and symptoms; in the way that they define pain and symptoms; and in the extent to which they seek help, make claims on others, and adjust their schedules to accommodate illness.

In understanding the individual's perception of illness, it is important to recognize that illness does not lend itself to rigid definition. The individual continually evaluates and re-evaluates the severity of symptoms in various situations.[3] Illness behavior involves an attempt to make sense of symptoms and to cope with them.[2] The evaluative and coping processes, and the decisions that result from them, may be limited by the individual's intelligence, as well as by his or her social and cultural understanding.[2,4]

The pharmacist who provides pharmaceutical care must think in terms of the patient's illness rather than the medically defined sickness condition. The patient's perception of his illness in this sense can affect his attitude and behavior in relation to using the medication. Consider that when a patient is receiving a prescription for an antibiotic, he is not just a case of "strep throat," but rather an individual who is experiencing discomfort swallowing, who has had to take the day off from work, and who wants some sympathy from his family. Likewise, when dispensing refill prescriptions, the pharmacist should consider that a patient's perceptions of his illness may be changing so that his original lack of concern about a sore throat has now become worry over the implications of a longer term condition, concern over being off work longer than expected, and possibly questions about the physician's and pharmacist's abilities to treat the condition.

Theories of Health-Related Behavior

Health-related behavior has been the subject of considerable research and theorizing in recent years. A full discussion of the existing literature is beyond the scope of this book, but for those interested in further study, the references provided for this chapter will be helpful. Theories pertaining to health-related behavior were developed primarily to understand the failure among patients to comply with medical treatments and to follow preventive health measures, such as immunization and regular health examinations.[5]

A variety of models has been constructed to help explain such behaviors.[2] One such model—the Health Belief Model—contains elements that are also found in many of the others, and therefore it will be used here as the basis of a discussion of the general concept of health-related behavior. Figure 3.1 illustrates this model.

The Health Belief Model suggests that the likelihood that an individual will take action in the interest of his or her health depends largely on that person's perception of the threat posed by a particular disease.[6] For example, patients who believe that high blood pressure may result in a heart attack are thought to be more likely than others to take their high blood pressure medication, watch their diet, exercise, and have regular physical checkups.

The perception of the threat of disease, however, depends on many factors, including so-called modifying factors, individual perceptions, and triggers to action.[6] Modifying factors can include a host of variables ranging from the demographic (age, gender, race, ethnicity, etc.) and the socio-psychological

Figure 3.1
The Health Belief Model

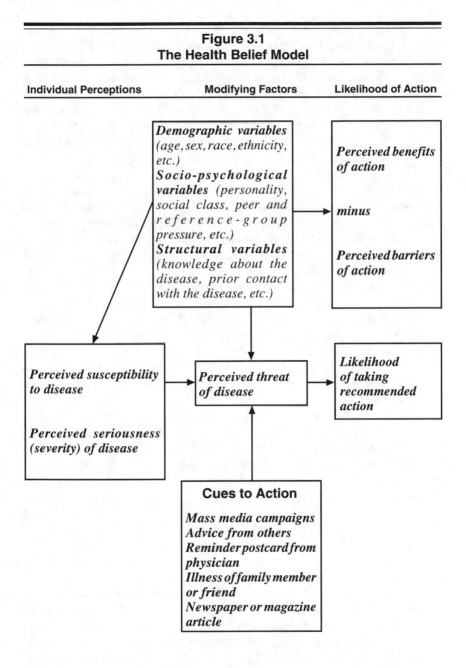

Individual Perceptions   **Modifying Factors**   **Likelihood of Action**

Demographic variables (age, sex, race, ethnicity, etc.)
Socio-psychological variables (personality, social class, peer and reference-group pressure, etc.)
Structural variables (knowledge about the disease, prior contact with the disease, etc.)

Perceived benefits of action

minus

Perceived barriers of action

Perceived susceptibility to disease

Perceived seriousness (severity) of disease

Perceived threat of disease

Likelihood of taking recommended action

Cues to Action

Mass media campaigns
Advice from others
Reminder postcard from physician
Illness of family member or friend
Newspaper or magazine article

Source: Becker MH, Rosenstock IM. Compliance with medical advice. In: eds. Steptoe A, Mathews A. Health Care and Human Behaviour. London: Academic Press, 1984.

(personality, social class, peer and reference-group pressure, etc.) to the structural (knowledge about the disease, prior contact with the disease, etc.). For example, a young, sexually active girl who is cautious by nature, knows about birth-control methods, and has a friend who became pregnant, may perceive that the chances of becoming pregnant are high. She is therefore very likely to use birth control.

Individual perceptions of the seriousness of a disease and of personal susceptibility to that disease may also affect a person's perception of its threat. For example, an individual may believe that high blood pressure is not a serious disease at all, and that it is unlikely to have a life-threatening effect.

Individual perceptions are determined, to a degree, by modifying factors.[6] For example, an individual whose parents lived to a very old age and who believes that any serious illness should have some obvious symptoms may believe that his family is not very susceptible to heart disease and that his diagnosed high blood pressure is not very serious. Therefore, he may not consider his condition to be much of a threat and may consequently fail to take his medication or follow advice about diet and regular checkups.

External factors can also affect an individual's perception of the threat of a disease and act as a trigger to action. Articles or campaigns in the media, advice from others, and similar illness among family members or friends may constitute triggers to action.[6] For example, reports in the media about the spread of an influenza virus, combined with reports of numerous deaths from the flu among the elderly population, might trigger the perception in elderly individuals that influenza poses a real threat to them, and lead them to get influenza vaccinations.

Even though the perceived threat of disease may be high, an individual may still fail to take action because of various factors that limit his or her ability to do so; in other words, because the perceived barriers to action outweigh the perceived benefits of action.[6] For example, an individual who has difficulty paying for his high blood pressure medication may fail to take it regularly, even though he believes that it would be beneficial to do so.

In a review of 46 studies involving the health belief model, Janz and Becker found that barriers to action represented the most important variable in explaining health-related behavior. This was followed in descending order of importance, by perception of susceptibility, benefits of action, and perception of seriousness or severity of the condition.[7]

Interestingly, the findings of studies exploring preventive-health behavior are significantly different from those of studies that seek to explain noncompliance. This suggests that certain variables are more important in some situations than in others.[6] In addition, studies involving patients in various age groups, with differing medical conditions find different factors to be important.[8] Perhaps the most important outcome of this research is the recognition that health-related behavior is extremely complicated and involves many variables – not just an individual's knowledge or personality.

For the pharmacist, this means that each counseling situation must be approached with an open mind with respect to the way the patient may be feeling about his or her illness and about medication use. Together, pharmacist and patient must explore the factors that are involved in the patient's individual situation, and determine which might be most important. For example, a patient whose job involves driving a truck will be concerned about the barriers to taking his prescribed medication regularly—he won't want to risk possible drowsiness on the job and may not have the opportunity to take regular doses. Another patient may think that there is not much point in taking his high blood pressure medication because he isn't very concerned about this condition and doesn't believe that the medication will do much good anyway.

How People Feel about Being Ill

Another important aspect of illness that pharmacists need to consider when dealing with a patient is the individual's emotional reactions to illness. Although people seek help for symptoms for a variety of reasons, they are most often prompted by concern about the potential seriousness of their symptoms or by the disruption of their normal ability to function, or both. In some cases, the symptoms and the series of events leading up to seeking and receiving help can arouse strong feelings. If pharmacists are able to recognize and understand these emotions, they will be able to interact and help patients more effectively. The range of emotions that may be experienced by individuals can include frustration, fear and anxiety, feelings of damage, anger, dependency, guilt, depression, and loss of self-esteem.[9,10] These feelings may occur to varying degrees in different people and in different situations, and may be encountered in patients receiving medications for even the most minor conditions, such as hemorrhoids or acne.

Frustration

It isn't difficult to understand the frustration associated with being ill. Most people have a routine in their lives, which is disrupted, to various degrees, by being ill. Perhaps the least of the disruptions is taking the time to visit the physician, and then the pharmacy. Frustration results from having to delay usual activities, as well as from unfamiliar restrictions, such as the inability to perform simple actions—for example, walking a certain distance or even laughing without pain or discomfort. The patient may also feel frustrated by the loss of certain pleasures, such as eating a highly spiced gourmet meal or enjoying sexual activities.[9] Frustration may result from the treatment for the condition if it results in loss of pleasure also for example not being allowed to drink alcohol because of an interaction with the medication.[9]

Such frustrations may manifest themselves in the patient's anger or impatience toward the pharmacist or in noncompliance, or both.[10] Although pharmacists cannot counteract the causes of these frustrations, they can encourage patients to find alternative pleasures and ways to minimize the inconvenience of delaying routine activities. They can also encourage patients, where appropriate, to resume as much of their normal activities as possible.[9]

Fear and Anxiety

Patients may experience feelings of fear as a result of real or imagined problems relating to their illness.[9,10] They may fear the physical outcome of their disease (pain, disfigurement, death, or long-term disability); the worsening of symptoms (e.g., more severe pain or permanent disability); or the social consequences of the illness (e.g., the shock, disgust, or fear experienced by friends or family; embarrassment; loss of employment).

Although fear is often apparent in the patient's physical appearance and manner (nervousness, pallor, and perspiration), it can also be less obvious and more difficult to detect. The patient may report physical symptoms such as stomach upsets, diarrhea, headaches, raised blood pressure and muscular tension. Fear can also manifest itself in the patient's behavior—in the nervous repetition of questions, the demand for attention, and the need for reassurance.

When the pharmacist perceives that fear is present, he can help the patient by making it clear he recognizes and accepts these feelings and by encouraging the patient to discuss them. The pharmacist may also be able to help alleviate certain fears by explaining symptoms and their possible outcomes, and by putting such fears into proper perspective. Reassurance can be given where appropriate, and aid in terms of referral to self-help groups or counseling may also be offered.[9]

Feelings of Damage

Another emotion sometimes aroused by illness is a feeling of damage.[9] This emotion may occur not only in illnesses where disfigurement or paralysis is evident, but in association with other illnesses as well. Patient's may perceive themselves to be impaired or "different" in some way, simply because their body is no longer functioning in its normal capacity. The patient's image of himself and his body has been damaged.[9]

By recognizing this emotion and by allowing the patient the opportunity to discuss it, the pharmacist may be able to help the patient come to terms with the feeling and, possibly, to see ways of resolving it.

Anger, Dependency, Guilt

A patient's experience of his illness is affected by his background of emotional reactions to previous illnesses and by patterns of behaving and coping developed during his lifetime.[9] Emotions such as anger, dependence, and guilt are expressed during illness primarily as a result of previous life experiences.[9]

Feelings of anger by the patient may or may not be verbalized. If such feelings are verbalized, they may be disruptive and upsetting to all; if they are not, they may still result in destructive behavior by the patient.[9] The pharmacist must recognize that anger shown by the patient, for example, while waiting for a prescription, may simply be the result of frustration as discussed above. This would best be dealt with by the pharmacist discussing the cause of anger with the patient.

As a result of their life experiences, patients sometimes become very dependent during illness, or alternatively refuse to become dependent at all.[9] Although dependence is necessary to a degree during severe illness, patients should be encouraged to become self-dependent.

For various personal reasons, patients may also feel guilt regarding their illness, or an inability to function normally.[9] Patients who experience guilt may appear passive and tolerant, communicate minimally, and appear withdrawn. Again, the pharmacist will need to discover if the patient's passivity is a result of guilt, and let the patient know that he recognizes, accepts, and understands such feelings.

Depression and Loss of Self-Esteem

When the emotions discussed above are allowed to continue without relief, they may progress to feelings of depression and loss of self-esteem.[9] Depression is recognizable by withdrawal and unwillingness to talk, eat, or engage in activity. Pharmacists should deal with depression by being aware of it and by directing the patient to professional psychological help.[9]

Self-esteem is a combination of a person's values, attitudes, and assumptions about herself or himself.[9] Prolonged or severe illness and the resulting dependency on others can result in loss of self-esteem. This is more difficult for the pharmacist to recognize, but may be apparent by the patient's acceptance of illness and an attitude of defeat. Again, the pharmacist should be alert to identifying this feeling and should recommend additional help. There are also some ways that pharmacists can help to improve a patient's self-esteem. For example, pharmacists can allow patients to have some feeling of control over their illness or treatment (e.g., showing them how to monitor symptoms, allowing them to decide whether they want a tablet or liquid, twice or four-times-daily dosage). The pharmacist can further improve the patient's self-esteem by showing the patient that he is concerned and interested in him.

Feelings Connected with Death and Dying

The most extreme and difficult situation that the pharmacist must deal with is one involving a dying patient and his family. Health professionals often try to avoid such situations, because they don't know how to react to the patient. In addition, the situation arouses in the pharmacist his own fears associated with death as well as frustration at not being able to prevent the patient's death and suffering.[11]

In a pioneering study, Kübler-Ross observed dying patients and identified five stages that the terminally ill patient may go through.[12] Not all patients progress through each stage in the same order, and some may remain in one stage or even repeat stages. The five stages, as described in Table 3.1, are denial, anger, bargaining, depression, and acceptance.

Denial is a common first reaction for patients to go through on discovering they have a terminal illness. This is a kind of self-protective mechanism during which the patient copes with the situation by questioning the diagnosis even after a second opinion, or simply dismisses the prognosis. Although the patient is trying to assimilate information about his or her illness, the patient may need information to be repeated by the pharmacist. The pharmacist should not attempt to convince the patient of the truth of the situation, and should be prepared to be understanding of the patient's point of view and simply listen.

When coping with terminal illness, patients may become angry, and express anger toward various people and objects. They may blame, question, challenge and continually complain, often driving people away so that they become lonely. The pharmacist should try not to take the anger personally. He should listen, allow the patient to vent his feelings, and try to empathize.

Patients often try to accept their situation by bargaining with caregivers and with God for more time. Again the pharmacist should be prepared to listen, but may also help by trying to focus on the possible rather than the impossible.

Because of the hopelessness of the illness and treatment, imminent separation from loved ones, and loss of contact with the outside world, terminally ill patients often become depressed. The patient is grieving and may become silent or often cry. The pharmacist should provide privacy, but be prepared to listen and encourage sharing of feelings if the patient wishes.

Some patients reach an acceptance of their situation, during which they seem ready to die. They may appear devoid of feelings, but are not bitter. They may wish to be alone with loved ones only. The pharmacist should honor this wish for privacy, and offer help where appropriate in dealing with unfinished business.

Pharmacists can help their patients and their patients' families by recognizing these stages and dealing with them accordingly. Suggestions for communicating with a dying patient will be discussed in Chapter 8.

How People Feel about Taking Medication

From the medical perspective discussed in the previous chapter, patients take medication because it has been prescribed and because they have been advised by a medical authority to do so. From the helping perspective, however, we recognize that patients take medication for a variety of reasons. In order to help patients get the most benefit from their medication, the pharmacist must learn to view medication use from the patient's perspective.

Patients may have a variety of personal reasons for taking medication[13]. In a study of anticonvulsant users, the reason most commonly given was practical. Patients saw medication use as a fact of life, necessary if seizures were to be controlled and, social and personal disruptions avoided. The second was psychological—to reduce worry. The third reason was the desire to ensure "normality," in the sense of leading a "normal life" without seizures.

In addition, for these individuals, using medication was not only a part of everyday life, but became a sign of illness, symbolizing, to themselves and others,

Table 3.1   Stages of Dying and How the Pharmacist Can Help

Stage	Patient Behavior	How the Pharmacist Can Help
Denial *"No, not me"*	*A self-protective reaction mechanism in response to the initial shock* *Patient may dismiss or question the diagnosis even after it has been confirmed by a second opinion*	*Understand, listen* *May need to repeat information since patient may not absorb it all* *Do not try to convince*
Anger *"Why me?"*	*Anger toward people and objects* *May blame, question and challenge, envying those who are well* *Feeling of helplessness* *Often complains continually and drives others away, thus becoming lonely*	*Try not to get angry in return* *Don't just take the anger but try to find out why the patient is angry* *Let patient vent feelings* *Listen* *Empathize, recognize that the patient is not angry with you*
Bargaining *"Yes, me— but..."*	*Tries to accept the situation* *Tries to bargain with God and people for more time*	*Listen* *Help patient focus on what is possible, rather than on the impossible*
Depression *"Yes, me"*	*Realizes the truth and now grieves and mourns* *May be very silent; may cry*	*Allow patient to express sorrow* *Allow privacy, but listen if patient wants to talk*
Acceptance *"I'm ready"*	*No longer angry or depressed* *Not bitter resignation, but a need to deal with unfinished business* *May separate himself from others and wish to be with only one loved person by his side*	*Allow for privacy*

Adapted from Jang R. Emotional reaction to illness and treatment. In: Communication Skills in Patient Counseling on OTC Drugs. Chapel Hill, N.C.: Health Sciences Consortium, 1980: Kübler-Ross E. What is it like to be dying? American Journal of Nursing. 1971;71(1):54-60; Okolo N, McReynolds J. Counseling the terminally ill. Am Pharm.1987;27(9):37-40.

that they were different and, perhaps, inferior.

Patients are also constantly making independent decisions about whether to take their medication and about the manner in which they will do so.[14] When patients are given information and advice from health professionals, they make decisions to modify their health behaviors by considering new information in light of previously held information, experiences, beliefs, and biases.[14]

Bias affects the way patients acquire and process information during the decision making process. For example, patients don't always gather information from all sides before making a decision, and some patients decide that the information they have gathered does not necessarily apply in their particular case.

In addition, patients have difficulty processing large amounts of "probablistic information," such as the chances of side effects occurring or the consequences that could arise if their condition were to continue unchecked.

Most importantly, it has been found that patients' decision-making processes are not always logical. Pharmacists need to understand this decision-making process and be nonjudgmental about the illogical ways that people make decisions.

Considering Health-Related Quality of Life

When we consider how patients feel about being ill and taking medication, we should also take into consideration the effects of illness and medication on the patient's *quality of life* (QOL). This concept takes into account a person's physical, emotional, mental, and intellectual capacity; his ability to function at work, in social situations, and within the family; his perception of his abilities; and satisfaction with those abilities.[15]

Health-care policy makers, pharmaceutical companies, third-party payers, and the Food and Drug Administration are beginning to take quality of life into consideration when evaluating pharmaceuticals.[15]

Assessment of the impact of illness and medication use on a patient's quality of life is complex. Patrick and Erickson define QOL as "the value assigned to the duration of life as modified by the social opportunities, perceptions, functional states, and impairments that are influenced by disease, injuries, treatments, or policy."[15] Unfortunately pharmacists don't have access to all this information when talking with patients, but some of it can be illuminated through discussion.

In terms of pharmaceutical care, we must consider the patient's quality of life when we identify and prioritize medication-related problems, determine treatment goals, and develop monitoring protocols. For example, when we consider outcomes of treatment, we should realize that measures such as sedimentation rate or blood pressure mean little to the patient, but that physical discomfort, the ability to walk briskly up the stairs, and financial impact have real-world significance. We can realize that a patient taking antihypertensive medication may perceive that his quality of life has actually been reduced because of unpleasant side effects, reduced feeling of well-being, increased medical expenses, and restricted activities. This may result in noncompliance, reduced confidence in physician and pharmacist, as well as worsening of medical condition because of a negative outlook. The physician however may see blood pressure reduced and consider therapy to be a success.[15]

Pharmacists have the opportunity to anticipate such quality of life effects and help the patient and physician take them into consideration in selecting and evaluating therapy. Some suggestions of how the pharmacist can contribute are listed in Table 3.2.

Table 3.2   Pharmacist's Contribution to Quality of Life Consideration

1. Discuss with the patient whether the therapy is likely to interfere with important aspects of his or her lifestyle

2. Explain to the patient what he or she can and cannot expect from therapy and help the patient weigh the benefits against costs

3. Offer suggestions on how to minimize the impact of negative effects of therapy on the patient's QOL

4. Be prepared for medication-induced patient complaints

5. Communicate medication-related QOL complaints to the physician and suggest alternatives

6. Include lifestyle characteristics such as hobbies and occupation on the patient's medication profile

Adapted from Smith M, Juergens J, Jack W. Medication and the Quality of Life. Am. Pharm. 1991;NS31(4):27-33.

Summary

This chapter has touched on the very complicated area of health and illness theory. These findings about patients' feelings and beliefs regarding illness and taking medication seem to suggest at least one thing very clearly: that simply telling patients to take their medication, or simply providing information about the medication, will not necessarily result in patient compliance—the subject of the next chapter.

References

1. Chappell N. Strain L, Blandford A. Health status and aging. In: Aging and Health Care: A Social Perspective. Toronto: Holt, Rinehart & Winston. 1986.

2. Mechanic D. Illness behavior. In: Medical Sociology. 2d ed. New York: Free Press. 1978.

3. Alonzo A. Everyday illness behavior: A situational approach to health status deviations. Soc Sci Med. 1979;13A:397-404.
4. Rakowski W. Health psychology and late life: The differentiation of health and illness for the study of health-related behaviors. Research on Aging. 1984;6(4):593-620.
5. Cummings KM, Becker MH, Maile MC. Bringing the models together: An empirical approach to combining variables used to explain health actions. J Behav Med. 1980;3(2):123-145.
6. Becker MH, Rosenstock IM. Compliance with medical advice. In: Health Care and Human Behaviour, eds Steptoe A, Mathews A. London: Academic Press. 1984.
7. Janz N, Becker MH. The health belief model: A decade later. Health Educ Q. 1984;11(1):1-47.
8. Owens N. Patient noncompliance: Subset analysis. Drug Topics. 1992;Supp 136(13):11-15.
9. Bernstein L, Bernstein RS. Emotions in illness and treatment. In: Interviewing: A Guide for Health Professionals. 4th ed. New York: Appleton-Century-Crofts. 1985.
10. Jang R. Emotional reactions to illness and treatment. In Communication Skills in Patient Counselling on OTC Drugs. Chapel Hill, NC: Health Sciences Consortium. 1980.
11. Okolo N, McReynolds J. Counseling the terminally ill. Am Pharm. 1987; 27(9):37-40.
12. Kübler-Ross E. What is it like to be dying? Am J Nurs. 1971;71(1):54-60.
13. Conrad P. The meaning of medication: Another look at compliance. Soc Sci Med. 1985;20(1):19-37.
14. Dolinsky D. How do the elderly make decisions about taking medications? J Soc Admin Pharm. 1989;6(3):127-37.
15. Smith M, Juergens J, Jack W. Medication and the quality of life. Am Pharm. 1991;NS31(4):27-33.

4
UNDERSTANDING
NONCOMPLIANCE

While preparing a refill prescription for a beta-blocker for an elderly patient, a pharmacist notes from the patient record that the previous quantity of medication would have lasted only 30 days, and it has now been 40 days since the prescription was dispensed. She plans to discuss this with the patient, since she knows about the possible serious implications of suddenly stopping beta-blockers, and of the long-term results of uncontrolled high blood pressure. As a responsible and concerned pharmacist, she is well aware of the issue of compliance.

Compliance has been defined as "the extent to which a person's behavior (in terms of taking medications, following diets, or executing lifestyle changes) coincides with medical or health advice."[1] As noted in Chapter 1, failure to comply is an enormous problem. Noncompliance has been designated by the National Council on Patient Information and Education as "America's other drug problem."[2] In a 1992 survey conducted by Schering Laboratories, 19% of patients admitted not following prescription directions exactly and 8.7% admitted not filling initial prescriptions.[3] However, self-reports of compliance can be expected to underestimate the problem. Depending on the group being studied, the type of medication, and various other factors, studies find noncompliance rates with drug therapy range from 13% to 93% with an average rate of 40%.[2] A range of noncompliance occurs, with an estimated one third of patients taking all of their prescribed medication, one third taking some of the prescription, and the final third not taking any of it.[4]

The outcome of noncompliance should be of utmost concern to pharmacists who wish to provide pharmaceutical care. Pharmaceutical care requires the identification, resolution, and prevention of drug-related problems, three of which pertain to noncompliance: 1) taking or receiving too little of the correct drug, 2) taking or receiving too much of the correct drug, 3) not taking or receiving the drug prescribed.[5] The concept of pharmaceutical care further requires the pharmacist to take responsibility for the outcome of medication use. Noncompliance results in a number of undesirable outcomes including prolonging or worsening of the medical condition; hospital and nursing home admissions; and in the extreme case, death.[5] In addition, the incalculable effects of noncompliance complicate the evaluation and approval of new pharmaceutical agents at the clinical investigations stage where optimum dosing is determined; and at the postapproval stage where unanticipated problems with dosing and side effects are monitored.[6] Finally, there is an enormous cost to society and the health care system , not only costs of treating the harmful results of noncompliance, but also costs of wasted medication and lost work days.[4]

The statistics on noncompliance are at once alarming and discouraging to health professionals. In the past, health professionals have often shown little interest in noncompliance, either appearing to trust blindly that their instructions were being followed, or accepting the reality of noncompliance and expecting little from patients. In fact, the state of the art of prescribing was summarized in 1975 by Charney: "the physician will be expected to prescribe with only approximate accuracy, and the patient will be expected to comply with only modest fidelity."[7]

Present times require health professionals to take a more enlightened approach to noncompliance. In light of pharmacists' newly recognized responsibility to effect outcomes of treatment, it becomes important for pharmacists to understand the factors that contribute to noncompliance and to employ techniques and approaches to overcome it.

Noncompliance Versus Self-Regulation

As a starting point in understanding the issue of noncompliance, it might be useful to consider the concept of "compliance." The word *compliance* itself suggests the medical-model approach: the patient must follow the physician's orders and "comply" with his or her directions.[1,8,9] Patients who do not "comply" are considered deviant. In fact, the dictionary definition of "compliance" is "yielding to the wishes of others."[10] This way of thinking implies that there is no place for the patient in decision making about drug use.

Also implicit in the definition of "compliance" is the notion that following the recommended advice is always correct and in the patient's best interest. There is an assumption that the condition being treated has been properly diagnosed; that the treatment is appropriate and effective, and does more good than harm; and that the prescribed regimen is understandable and achievable (i.e., directions are simple, dosing is convenient, cost and side effects are acceptable).[7] Patients, however, often do recover without having rigidly adhered to their physician's directions, and, conversely, prescribed treatments are not always effective—some "compliant" patients do not recover and some even get worse. In addition, drugs are on occasion prescribed unnecessarily or simply in an attempt to placate the patient.[11] In fact, reduction or discontinuance of medication may be warranted when in cases where unpleasant side effects and possibly dangerous adverse effects occur, often referred to as "intelligent noncompliance."[6] Such facts certainly challenge the premise on which the notion of compliance is based.[8,11]

Rather than considering the issue in terms of "noncompliance," we should see it from the perspective of "self-regulation" or, at least, "non-adherence."[1,8,9] From this patient-centered perspective, patients are seen to be active agents in their treatment. We must therefore look to the broader perspective of patients' lives to learn what makes them assume "self-regulation" in their medication regimens.[9]

Causes of Medication Self-Regulation (Noncompliance)

The pharmacist mentioned at the beginning of this chapter wondered why the patient was late for her refill prescription and what would cause her to be noncompliant. A number of theoretical models have been proposed to help us understand the phenomenon of noncompliance, and many different factors have been considered as contributors to noncompliance.[12-15] Studies have been conducted to explore factors contributing to noncompliance and suggestions have been made as to how we can better understand and deal with the noncompliant patient.[12-15] Together, these models and the findings of many studies indicate that the main contributing factors to noncompliance can be identified in the patient's health beliefs, the nature of communication between the patient and health professionals, and various psychological factors.[9]

Health Belief Factors Affecting Compliance

A number of factors included in the Health Belief Model discussed in the previous chapter may contribute to noncompliance. These factors include gender, race, age, education, cost of therapy, side effects, patient income, complexity of treatment regimens, and severity of disease.[15] Other theories suggest that patients will modify their compliant behavior based on logical thought into the risks of the disease and benefits of the treatment, with various internal and external factors modifying these thoughts.[15] A number of the factors suggested in these models and theories have been found to be significantly related to compliance.

The individual's perception of the seriousness of his or her condition has been found to be associated with noncompliance.[8] In a study of patients taking a short-term antibiotic regimen, compliers perceived their condition to be worse than did noncompliers.[16] An individual may not believe that his condition is sufficiently serious to warrant attention or may even deny that a problem exists. This often occurs in the case of psychiatric disorders, where the illness may compromise the patient's perceptions of threat.[2] The immediate threat of problems if medication is not taken appears to be significant. Patients taking anticonvulsants were found to be more likely to be compliant than those on antihypertensives.[17] Perception of the condition may relate to more personal values of treatment, for example, isotretinoin, used for cosmetic reasons of acne treatment, was found to be more likely to be complied with than antihypertensive drugs.[17]

The individual's perception of the efficacy of a prescribed treatment has also been found to be a relevant factor in compliance.[8] Patients may believe that no medication can alleviate their particular condition, or they may misunderstand the manner in which a medication is intended to help and therefore interpret it to be ineffective. For example, a medication such as amitriptyline may not exhibit an effect for several weeks during which time the patient, seeing little or no change, may come to believe that the drug is ineffective.

Another factor influencing compliance is the effect of family and friends (social support). In one study, although 43% of patients on antihypertensive therapy reported feeling better, only 1% of companions reported improvement, and 99% reported worsening of the patient's condition due to the patient's decreased energy, increased irritability, impaired memory, and enhanced hypochondriasis.[7] These companions may serve to deter medication-taking behavior.[7]

Other belief and behavioral factors found to be associated with compliance involve barriers to medication use, such as difficulties in following the prescribed regimen.[8] The more complex the regimen, the less compliant patients are likely to be. Many studies have found that as the number of required doses increases compliance decreases: once daily being most complied with, twice or three times daily dosing being equally poor compared to once daily, and four times daily being least complied with.[16,17] Difficulties in remembering to take medication several times daily or in fitting medication use into a daily routine have been suggested as reasons for this reduction in the likelihood of compliance.[16]

Therapy of a longer duration is also less likely to be complied with. This may result from the patient's difficulties in remembering and in scheduling doses. Decreasing compliance over time may also involve decreasing concern with the condition, or attempts to test the need for continued medication.[9]

The presence of adverse effects or side effects has also been found to reduce compliance, due to discomfort or fear of more serious effects, or both.[3,18] This may be particularly true if the patient has not been warned about the chance of side effects or has not been given suggestions about how to minimize such effects. In a survey of patients regarding the perception of risk of drugs, 90% of patients believed that precaution and warning information about a prescription would encourage them to take the drug exactly as prescribed.[19] Apparently, it is not simply the occurrence of adverse effects that interferes with compliance, but rather difficulty with particular adverse effects that the patient cannot tolerate or manage.[2]

In most studies conducted to date, no consistent relationship has been found to exist between compliance and demographic factors such as social class, age, gender, education, or marital status.[8,16] In addition, low intelligence, poor memory, or personality disorders have not been found to be related to noncompliance.[14]

Communication Factors

Various factors involved in the communication between the patient and health professional have been considered for their effects on compliance.[15] It has been suggested that if a message from a health professional is sent, received, comprehended, retained, and believed by a patient then the result will be compliance. Various factors affecting the communication process may affect compliance such as reinforcing information, cuing, and verbal and written communication.[15]

Noncompliance has been associated with minimal medical supervision, whereas higher compliance rates have been found to occur when patients are given explicit and appropriate instructions, more and clearer information, and more and better feedback.[9]

However, the effectiveness of the patient–health professional interaction appears to reside less in the improvement of the patient's knowledge than in the way that patient education is approached. To be most effective, the interaction has to involve strategies that modify the patient's health beliefs and attitudes.[11]

In addition to the factual content of the patient–health professional encounter, its emotional content has also proven to be relevant in matters of compliance—essentially, the lower the patient's satisfaction with the interaction, the greater the likelihood of noncompliance.[14] Studies of patient–physician interactions suggest that noncompliance is higher when patients find their physician unfriendly or when their expectations of their physician are not met.[9] In one study, non-compliers were judged to be less assertive, and less friendly during consultation with their physician than compliers.[16] In another study involving acceptance of nonprescription drug advice from a pharmacist, patients were more likely to follow the advice when the pharmacist was introverted rather than extraverted in personality.[20] The researchers suggested that patients may have perceived extraverted pharmacists as overbearing, unreliable, or untrustworthy.

Further evidence of the importance of satisfaction with pharmacist and physician was found in a recent survey of patients. A high percentage of patients who failed to take the proper dosage, did not take medication at proper times, or did not take the medication for the full duration found fault with the medication in some way. However, the perception that the medication failed was found to be partially related to dissatisfaction with the health professional interaction, since patients who reported being dissatisfied with the pharmacist's instructions and with the doctor's counsel were more likely to report that their medication failed.[3]

Simply interacting with the patient can make a difference in the case of the pharmacist–patient situation. Noncompliance was reduced by 25% when the pharmacist, rather than the clerk handed the medicine to the patient.[3]

Concern for the patient by the health-care professional and involvement by the patient in decisions regarding therapy also improve compliance.[2]

These findings suggest that if compliance is to be improved, the encounter must provide the patient with significantly more than simply factual information, but must also include emotional aspects.

Psychological Factors

In addition to health beliefs and communication factors, various psychological factors have been found to affect compliance.

Compliance is a type of behavior, and therefore, behavioral learning theories have been suggested to help find ways to explain and modify noncompliance.[15] In this regard, the provision of cues, rewards, contracts, and social support have been suggested methods to improve compliance.[15]

Patients' cognitive abilities may also affect their compliance with medication: patients formulate action plans, appraise the plans, and find ways to cope. They use their cognitive skills and emotional experiences to solve problems regarding their medication use, resulting in compliant or noncompliant behavior.[15]

Studies exploring the psychological factors involved in medication use point to the importance of the decision-making aspects of noncompliance, as well as to experiential learning. For example, noncompliance may be the result of an individual's decision to test the efficacy of the drug. In interviews of patients with epilepsy, Conrad found that patients often altered or discontinued their medication to test if it was having any effect and to determine whether they still had epilepsy.[9]

Experience may also be a positive aspect, in that experience taking medication on a regular basis may improve compliance. In one study, compliance improved as the number of concurrent medications increased.[17] The authors hypothesized that patients were forced to develop a dosage-administration strategy that ensured compliance.

An individual may also be noncompliant in an attempt to assert control – over the doctor-patient relationship or over the medical condition itself, especially if it is one that appears to be beyond control, such as epilepsy.[9] As discussed in Chapter 3, suffering from an illness, taking medication, and relying on health professionals can be perceived by the individual as increased dependence. Patients may attempt to regain that independence by means of altering their medication regimens.[9]

The patient's knowledge about the disease or the medication has not been shown to be directly related to compliance.[11] Knowledge is of limited value without the understanding or desire to apply it. There also is no evidence to suggest that a noncompliant *type* of individual exists.[8]

To summarize, studies have found that multiple factors are related to patient noncompliance, often working together within the same situation. The patient's perceptions and not the health professional's objective clinical judgement determine the evaluation of the seriousness of his condition or the complexity of his medication regimen.[16]

A summary of the factors that have been found to contribute to noncompliance is shown in Table 4.1.

Table 4.1   Causes of Medication Self-Regulation

Health Beliefs

>   *Perceived lack of seriousness of the disease and outcomes of*
>
>   *nontreatment*
>
>   *Perceived ineffectiveness of the treatment*
>
>   *Lack of social support*
>
>   *Complex medication regimens*
>
>   *Lengthy therapies*
>
>   *Presence of adverse effects*

Communication

>   *Low degree of medical supervision*

continued

Table 4.1   Causes of Medication Self-Regulation (continued)

Communication (continued)

> *Lack of instruction that is explicit, appropriate, clear, adequate in quantity, and including feedback*
>
> *Lack of strategies by health professional to modify attitudes and beliefs*
>
> *Low patient satisfaction in the interaction with the health professional*
>
> *Little or no interaction with health professional*
>
> *Health professional is perceived as unfriendly, lacking concern*
>
> *Health professional does not allow involvement of patient in decisions*

Psychological

> *Desire to test the efficacy of the drug*
>
> *Desire to assert control over the doctor–patient relationship, or even over a condition that appears to be beyond control.*
>
> *Lacking or negative experience with medication*

Approaches to Reducing Noncompliance

Equipped with this understanding of the factors that contribute to noncompliance, we can now consider ways in which the pharmacist can help to reduce noncompliance. Pharmaceutical care requires that pharmacists engage in a systematic and comprehensive process whereby they identify a patient's actual and potential drug-related problem; resolve the patient's actual drug-related problems; and prevent the patient's potential drug-related problems from becoming actual problems.[5] Approaches to improving compliance among patients will now be discussed as they relate to this.

Prevention of Potential Noncompliance

What can pharmacists do to encourage and assist their patients to be compliant? All patients should be viewed as potentially noncompliant.[2] As such, each situation must be considered individually in terms of the risks of noncompliance for this individual patient in this particular situation.

In developing a plan to prevent noncompliance, the pharmacist must pay attention to three aspects of patient counseling: 1) communication with the patient, 2) provision of information, and 3) strategies to prevent noncompliance.

Communication with the Patient

As discussed above, in order to prevent noncompliance, there must be communication with the patient. The pharmacist must engage the patient in discussion to establish a relationship with the patient. Further communication must occur to allow the pharmacist to proceed through the pharmaceutical care process to gather appropriate information determine methods to prevent noncompliance, and carry out these.[5]

A number of aspects of communication with the patient can help to prevent noncompliance:

1. *Patient Satisfaction with Communication:* The patient is more likely to be compliant if the physician and pharmacist engage in a conversation with the patient regarding his or her medication, and if the patient is satisfied with that communication.[3,14]

2. *Manner of the Communication:* The manner of the communication with the patient is of great importance and should not be coercive, frightening, threatening, or demeaning.[3] The pharmacist should not insist that the patient comply, but rather should offer the patient help with gaining the most benefit from his medication, convincing the patient that compliance would be in his own best interest. The pharmacist must not frighten the patient regarding possible adverse effects, or threaten him regarding the dangers of noncompliance.

3. *Nature of Communication*: In order to set this tone, the nature of the communication is important. It should involve not just presentation of information, but also discussion. The patient should be involved as much as possible in the interaction and in decisions regarding medication use (e.g. when to take, dosage form preferred). For example, a young teenager may have been prescribed an antibiotic in tablet form, but still prefer to use the liquid form used as a child. By discovering this through discussion, then arranging for the appropriate change in the prescription, the pharmacist would likely encourage the patient to take the medication to completion as instructed.

4. *Content of Communication:* The discussion with the patient should also include inquiry into the patient's perceptions of medication use. This can help the pharmacist determine the kinds of misperceptions that may be at play and the types of information and behavioral strategies that might be most beneficial for that patient.

   Even the patient who initially intends to comply will test the medication regimen for symptom relief, side effects, and inconvenience.[11] The patient will weigh the perceived costs and benefits of medication use and will adjust the degree of his compliance accordingly. It is therefore necessary for the pharmacist to discover some of the costs and benefits as perceived by the patient, and to address them before they occur. Directly asking the patient if he perceives any difficulties with taking the medication is therefore recommended.

   Once the patient's perceptions of drug use and potential problems relating to compliance have been identified, the pharmacist can proceed to address this through further discussion, provision of information, and specific strategies.

5. *Frequency of Communication:* The pharmacist should also encourage future communication by suggesting that the patient call to discuss any problems or concerns that arise in the future.

Since the patient's decision making about his illness and medication use is a continuous process, the pharmacist must follow the patient's progress and continue to interact with him after the initial prescription has been dispensed. A discussion with the patient during refill prescription counseling will allow the pharmacist to explore any changing beliefs and perceptions about the illness or medications that the patient may have developed since the first counseling session. This discussion will also allow the pharmacist to determine if any side effects are occurring that may become bothersome and lead to noncompliance. By dealing with any such problems, the pharmacist can continue to prevent noncompliance from developing.

6. *Method of Communication:* A combination of verbal and written communication is most likely to improve compliance and is preferred by patients.[2,15] The patient then has an opportunity to discuss information with the pharmacist in person, as well as review information provided at a later date to aid recall and to check information as it is needed (e.g., what to do about side effects when they occur). Many audiovisual materials are also available today. In addition, communication with the patient must be made clear by avoiding the use of jargon and by matching the patient's language and education levels as best as possible. These and other aspects of communication with patients and the use of various counseling aids will be discussed in further detail in Chapters 6 and 7.

Provision of Information

Through appropriate communication with the patient, the pharmacist is able to determine what type of information would best prevent noncompliance, and how best to present that information.

As has already been pointed out, simply providing information about medication use is of limited effectiveness. Although adequate information and clear instructions for use are obviously essential, they are not sufficient to encourage compliance.[8,11] A review of studies evaluating strategies for improving compliance found that providing information was shown to be effective in only slightly more than half of the studies.[12]

Providing information may however have some effect on attitudes and beliefs, and this may in turn have an effect on compliance.[12] In addition, the attention received by the patient in the course of instruction on medication use may contribute to improving compliance.

There are a number of factors concerning the provision of information that are important in preventing noncompliance:

1. *Persuasiveness:* It appears that the effectiveness of information provision

depends on the persuasiveness of the health professional's communication and on the extent of his or her attempts to motivate the patient.[8,9] Therefore, the method of information provision and communication techniques of the pharmacist are critical.

2. *Information Regarding Use:* Of course, in order to comply, a patient must always be provided with correct, appropriate, and complete instructions including how much medication to use, when to take it, how long to continue use including refill information, and what to do if a dose is missed.

3. *Information Regarding Illness and How and When Medication Will Help:* In addition, the patient needs information about his condition and the ways in which the medication is expected to help the condition. For example, a patient prescribed cimetidine for an ulcer needs to understand that an ulcer is a lesion in the stomach resulting in part from an excess of acid, and that the medication will help to reduce the amount of acid released in the stomach, allowing the ulcer to heal. This will hopefully prevent the patient from using the medication intermittently "as needed" rather than continually until the ulcer is healed.

   The patient should also be made aware of the amount of time it may take before pain and discomfort are reduced—in other words, when some effect of the medication is likely to be felt. This will help prevent any misperceptions on the patient's part about the seriousness of the condition or the effectiveness of the medication.

4. *Information About Side Effects:* Since the occurrence of side effects or fear of side effects occurring have been found to contribute to noncompliance, patients should be told about the signs of any common side effects that may occur. The provision of information about side effects and adverse effects reduces noncompliance by reducing fear and by allowing for a more appropriate handling of problems.[21,22] This positive effect may also arise out of the patient's greater sense of control over the effects of the medication. As mentioned above, patients report that such information would encourage them to be compliant.[9]

   Patients should also be told what they can do to prevent or minimize side effects. Signs of adverse effects should also be explained. The pharmacist should emphasize that these effects are very rare, but that it is nonetheless important to be able to recognize them as soon as they occur in order to allow for their early detection and management.

   Some pharmacists hesitate to discuss side effects and adverse effects with patients for fear that this may cause suggestible patients to later imagine that they are indeed experiencing the described effects. This, however, has not been found to be the case: studies have shown that patients who receive such information generally have no greater experience of side effects than those who do not.[23,24]

5. *Special Techniques*: Information regarding techniques to apply the medication if necessary, and ways to remember medication use should also be provided to reduce the chance of noncompliance due to difficulties following the regimen.
6. *Quantity and Level:* Information should not be too comprehensive or detailed for a patient to absorb or understand according to his or her education level, disabilities, or emotional state, since this may actually compromise rather than enhance compliance.[2] The specific types of information that can benefit patients, and the best ways to present such information, will be discussed in greater detail in Chapters 5, 6, and 7.

Strategies for Preventing Compliance

Since noncompliance is considered a behavior that is affected by beliefs, experience, etc., a variety of behavioral strategies are recommended to prevent noncompliance.[2,8,11,25] Such strategies may include the following:

1. Working with the physician to simplify medication schedules by reducing the number of drugs, reducing the number of daily dosage intervals, and adjusting the dosage regimen to better accommodate the patient's daily routine.
2. Supplying medication reminders and organizers, such as pill containers with alarms or organized compartments, and individualized drug-taking check-off charts.
3. Reminding patients by telephone or mail about their prescription refills.
4. Enlisting the support of the patient's spouse or other family members to remind and encourage the patient to take the prescribed medication.

These methods not only help to prevent incidents of noncompliance that arise out of practical difficulties in taking medication, but they also attempt to change individuals' attitudes or beliefs.

Identification of Noncompliance

When a patient comes to the pharmacy to pick up a refill prescription, the pharmacist has an opportunity to identify noncompliance. Identification of noncompliance requires the pharmacist to gather information to detect whether noncompliance is occurring; to ascertain the details of the noncompliance, its frequency and the situations that precipitate it; and to determine the factors that are contributing to noncompliance.

Detecting Noncompliance

The first clue to noncompliance may come from the patient record. If, according to the date that the prescription was last filled, the expected period for refill has been significantly exceeded, the pharmacist might conclude that noncompliance is occurring. Although serum levels or other clinical indicators may be a more precise check on compliance, refill records have been found to result in only about 10% higher apparent compliance than direct serum assay.[15]

The pharmacist should keep in mind, however, that noncompliance may not be the only explanation for an apparent late or early refill. Other reasons could be that the patient received verbal instructions from the physician to alter the dosage or had the prescription filled at a different pharmacy in the interim. Alternatively, noncompliance may not be apparent from the patient record. Patients sometimes continue to re-order medication on a regular basis, while stock-piling medication, possibly because they want their doctor to believe they are being compliant, or because in some cases the medication is being paid for by a third party and the patient feels they should "save it up" for a time when they may no longer receive such benefits. In addition, pill taking is often intermittent and random rather than systematic, and patients often omit or delay doses or miss a day or more at a time, but may make up for it just before a physician visit (known as "the white coat effect" or "toothbrush effect").[2,14] This irregular dosing may not be readily apparent from the patient's chart.[7]

The pharmacist must therefore interview the patient to determine if noncompliance is occurring as indicated on the chart or in the absence of chart evidence. This should be done with an open mind and with careful attention to the tone of the inquiry (i.e., *it should not sound like an inquisition*). Use of open-ended questions to encourage the patient to provide as much information as possible and gentle probing to determine when the medication is usually taken will help to determine the extent of noncompliance without alienating the patient.

Apart from refill counseling, noncompliance may come to the pharmacist's attention during a medication history interview conducted for a new patient. Techniques for the detection of noncompliance during medication history interviews will be discussed further in Chapter 5.

Noncompliance may also come to the pharmacist's attention through a comment or inquiry by the physician or patient regarding poor response to medication or the occurrence of side effects. These outcomes may be a result of improper use, for example, heart rhythm abnormalities resulting from inter-mittent use of beta-blockers.

In addition, pharmacists can detect noncompliance through sponsoring or becoming involved in "brown bag" programs such as that promoted by The National Council on Patient Information and Education.[4] Such programs encourage patients to put all their prescription and nonprescription medications in a bag and take them to an announced place where pharmacists and other health-care professionals review them. Pharmacists involved in these programs are ideally situated to discuss regular medication use with patients and to detect noncompliance.

On a more formal level, a compliance clinic may be conducted, where patients are seen regularly with the intent of assessing patient compliance through self-assessment by patients and through interviews by pharmacists.[26, 27]

Ascertaining the Details of Noncompliance

Once the pharmacist has found that noncompliance is indeed occurring, he can proceed to ascertain the details of the noncompliance. This will help the pharmacist to evaluate if indeed this is a serious problem to be reported to the physician (since it may be causing a poor response which may be misinterpreted by the physician) or rather it is a minor or temporary problem that can be corrected by the pharmacist and patient alone. This also assists the pharmacist in the pharmaceutical care process to list and rank the problems.

The pharmacist must probe to find out the details of frequency, duration, and degree of noncompliance and the situations that surround it. Noncompliance may be occurring only occasionally, as in the case of the patient who skips a dose when he goes to a party because he doesn't want to mix alcohol with his medication. Alternatively, noncompliance may be very frequent, as in the case of the patient who uses medication only for symptomatic relief rather than on a continual basis as prescribed for the prevention of symptoms. It may occur regularly at a certain time of day; for example, afternoon doses are always skipped on work days only.

Sensitivity in questioning the patient is important. General questions about any difficulties that the patient may be experiencing with the medication are likely to be most productive, inviting the patient to divulge problem situations. More specific questions can then follow to determine the relevant details. Suggested dialogues and further aspects of such probing will be discussed in Chapters 5 and 7, and Appendix B.

Determining Factors Contributing to Noncompliance

After ascertaining the details of noncompliance, the pharmacist must investigate the factors contributing to that noncompliance before attempting to resolve it.

Pharmacists often make erroneous assumptions about the reasons for noncompliance, particularly in assuming that patients simply forget to take their medication. In the previous section many possible reasons for noncompliance were suggested, and patients may exhibit one or a combination of these factors.

In the course of discussion, the pharmacist should be able to explore most of the possible factors involved in noncompliance, from health beliefs to patient–physician communication and psychological factors.

One way to approach evaluation is to focus on the patient, the medication, spouse/family/peers, and the patient–health professional relationship.[28]

1. *The Patient:* Factors such as the patient's knowledge, attitudes, values, and perceptions about their illness or therapy need to be investigated.[27,28] The pharmacist must determine whether the patient has become apathetic or frustrated about the treatment and whether the patient has lost confidence in the ability of the medication to treat his or her symptoms. If the patient has lost confidence, the pharmacist must determine why.

2. *The Medication:* Factors such as the skills of the patient and diffi-culty following a regimen need to be investigated, as well as the lack of availability of resources and services that could help the patient with compliance.[27,28] In particular, the pharmacist should focus attention on the medication regimen. Does it need to be simplified, in particular with regard to decreasing the number of daily doses? How can it be organized to coordinate better with the patient's daily routines? In addition, the pharmacist must determine whether side effects have emerged that might be discouraging the patient from using the medication. Is the patient reluctant to continue use because side effects are causing discomfort, because they are inconvenient, or because they cause fear?

3. *Spouse/Family/Peers:* Attitudes and behaviors of peers, family, and employers should be considered.[27,28] The pharmacist should pay attention to aspects of the patient's social life. Are family members or, possibly, friends involved in supporting compliance? If not, can they become more actively involved? Is the patient receiving any help with his medication?

4. *The Patient–Health Professional Relationship:* The patient's relation-ship with his/her physician, as well as with the pharmacist himself must also be explored by the pharmacist.[27,28] Has the patient become dissatisfied with some aspect of these relationships? Perhaps he/she has a personality conflict with one of his/her health professionals or feels a lack of confidence in the health professional's knowledge regarding his/her condition. On a more subtle level, the patient may simply feel powerless with regard to his/her own treatment.

Resolution of Noncompliance

Once noncompliance has been detected by the pharmacist, it is now his responsibility to resolve this problem. The pharmacist should proceed to identify the desired outcomes of his or her intervention, develop a plan, select strategies that motivate the patient, select various techniques and tools, then follow-up to insure that desired outcomes result.

Identifying the Desired Outcomes of a Plan to Resolve Noncompliance

As described in the pharmaceutical care process, once the patient's problems have been identified, the pharmacist should establish a desired pharmacotherapeutic outcome for each drug-related problem.[5] Depending on the factors that the pharmacist has determined to be contributing to the patient's noncompliance, the desired outcome of the pharmacist's action may be any one or all of the following:[5]

(a) The patient should receive the appropriate medication (e.g., requiring a medication change to improve the effectiveness, prevent side effects, or offer simpler dosing);

(b) The patient should receive the appropriate dose of a drug at the appropriate time and interval (e.g., a change in the dosage to a long acting medication to simplify dosing, or a change in the patient's beliefs and behavior regarding medication);

(c) Side effects the patient is experiencing should be removed (e.g., suggest taking medication with food to reduce stomach irritation).

The pharmacist also needs to specify how he or she will determine that the outcomes of actions to resolve noncompliance have been accomplished with respect to the following parameters:[5]

(a) Patient—a change in the patient can be identified, e.g. an improvement in a side effect symptom; an illness symptom; a quality of life variable; laboratory finding.

(b) Progress—for each patient indicator the degree of improvement is stated, e.g. patient will be able walk to the bus stop when desired; blood sugar will be within acceptable limits when tested regularly.

(c) Time—a time frame for achieving each outcome is stated (e.g. the patient will be able to walk to the bus stop after continuing on anti-inflammatory therapy regularly for 3 weeks).

The pharmaceutical care model also specifies that the plan should be documented.[5]

Developing a Plan to Resolve Noncompliance

Once the outcomes have been decided, the pharmacist must develop a plan to accomplish them. The plan should include: assessing needs; specifying goals and objectives; delineating content, strategies and resources; and evaluating the program.[27]

One important aspect of the plan to resolve noncompliance is the need for communication with the physician and other health-care workers. Any needed alterations in regimens and dosage forms to improve compliance must be negotiated with the prescribing physician. There is also a need for the pharmacist to advise the physician of regularly occurring noncompliance by a patient, since such behavior could be causing distortion in the physician's evaluation of the efficacy of the prescribed treatment. In addition, the physician and other health professionals, such as nurses and social workers, may be able to help formulate the plan aimed at resolving noncompliance. Disclosure to the physician should be discussed with the patient, in consideration of patient confidentiality. The pharmacist's interactions with other health professionals will be discussed further in Chapter 7.

When developing a plan for resolution of noncompliance, attention must again be drawn to the difference in the approaches associated with the medical model and the helping model. In accordance with the latter, the aim of treatment should *not* be to *make the patient comply*, but rather to *join with the patient* to overcome perceived problems relating to medication use. The pharmacist must convey to the patient an attitude that says, "I'm here to help you get the most benefit from your medication."

Armed with the information gathered during the process of indentification of noncompliance, the pharmacist, together with the patient and other health professionals, can proceed to select various strategies. These involve some of the strategies discussed above with respect to preventing noncompliance, as well as the educational approaches discussed in Chapter 2. The plan should include techniques to motivate the patient, as well as various interventions specific to overcoming that particular patient's problems with medication use. A summary of techniques to resolve compliance is shown in Table 4.2.

Strategies to Motivate the Patient

Motivation involves getting the patient's cooperation as a partner in attaining optimal therapy. Patients—particularly those who are not compliant— are often unwilling recipients of counseling. Patients may not expect to be counseled and may not have actually asked for help. Noncompliant patients may also feel embarrassed or guilty about their noncompliance and may therefore be reluctant to discuss the subject.

The "reluctant client" should be approached using strategies that will increase his or her readiness for counseling.[29] The reasons and goals of counseling should be explained to such a patient in an open and nonjudgmental way. Resistance may be also approached by asking the patient directly—but in a nonconfrontational manner—about his or her reluctance to comply.

Depending on the factors contributing to noncompliance in a patient, the pharmacist can motivate the patient through a variety of strategies: [2,30,31]

1. *Explain Benefits of Medication:* One method involves explaining how the medication will benefit the patient. The pharmacist should try to answer the patient's unspoken question, "What's in it for me?" This addresses health beliefs and misperceptions of susceptibility of the disease as well as misperceptions of the value of the medication that often affect compliance.

2. *Raise Awareness of Body Cues:* Another motivational method involves raising the patient's awareness of the body cues that signal the need for the medication. For example, a patient with high blood pressure might be shown how to take his own blood pressure and how to identify the initial high-level reading that registers before medication use.

3. *Explain Ways to Self-Evaluate:* Similarly, cues can be devised to help the patient to evaluate the outcome of therapy. For example, the pharmacist may encourage the patient to continue taking his own blood pressure on a regular basis, thus proving to himself that the medication effectively keeps his blood pressure down.

4. *Help Develop Coping Mechanisms:* The pharmacist can also help the patient develop coping mechanisms to deal with circumstances

that make it difficult to adhere to medication use. For example, if a patient is concerned about co-workers' reactions to his or her use of an anti-convulsant, the pharmacist might discuss the feared reactions and suggest ways for the patient either to broach the issue with his co-workers or to take the medication without others knowing (by means of alternative dosing, etc.).

These motivational methods have been found to be particularly effective for long-term medication use.[30] A combination of the appropriate motivational methods is generally more successful than one method alone.[2,15]

Selection of Techniques and Tools to Resolve Noncompliance

In addition to motivating noncompliant patients to adhere to medication regimens, pharmacists should provide patients with tools and techniques to aid compliance. A variety of tools and techniques, some of which were discussed, may be involved.[2,4,14]

1. *Compliance Aids:* A variety of compliance aids have been developed for pharmacists to offer to patients. These include special medication containers to remind patients when to administer doses; medication caps with timepieces, and alarms; pill reminder packages; compliance packaging that provides the patient with one treatment cycle in a ready-to-use package; calendars or drug-reminder charts to check off doses taken; telephone or mail reminders for refills.[2,4] These types of devices will be discussed further in Chapter 6.

2. *Enlisting Support:* Another technique the pharmacist can use to resolve noncompliance involves enlisting the support of the spouse, other family members, or members of the patient's support network to encourage and remind the patient to take medication. The pharmacist should investigate the views and perceptions of family members carefully, since they may have negative views of the treatment or condition and actually may be a cause of the noncompliance.[7] The pharmacist can try to gain the support of these individuals and suggest ways they can help with patient compliance, such as reminders to take medication and reassurance over the effectiveness of treatment and the need to treat the condition.

3. *Increase Supervision:* Shortening the intervals for refills may help to improve compliance by allowing the pharmacist to review medication use and to discuss this with the patient. This allows the pharmacist to detect problems that contribute to compliance over time such as the development of side effects; changes in social support; changes in attitudes and beliefs; changes in personal schedules, etc. Regular visits to the physician and personalized attention by the pharmacist and physician have been found to improve compliance.[7] In addition, follow-up counseling by telephone or in person can allow the pharmacist to discuss these issues with the patient.

4. *Social-Service Intervention:* Social-service intervention by means of a visiting nurse, a public-health nurse, a social worker, or a home-care worker may be recommended in certain cases to monitor and encourage the patient. This is particularly helpful where the patient has little or no social support, or where disabilities or cognitive deficits may be contributing to noncompliance.

5. *Alternative Dosing:* The pharmacist may need to recommend that the physician switch the patient to an alternative dosing schedule or dosage form (e.g., long acting medications, transdermal drug delivery system). Since most studies find more frequent and complicated dosing significantly increase noncompliance rates, this is a simple remedy that should be considered in many cases. However, long-acting medications may not be appropriate in all patients or conditions, particularly where toxic levels may accumulate, or where variations in dosing may be needed.

6. *Behavioral Modification Techniques:* Since many of the factors contributing to noncompliance involve a patient's beliefs and behavior, behavioral modification techniques should be considered to resolve noncompliance problems. Drawing up a "contract" between the patient and the health professional that spells out behavioral expectations, incentives, and rewards for compliance has been used successfully in some situations.[2] Through this technique, the patient is assisted by having the specific behavior outlined, by being involved in the decision-making process, by making a formal commitment, and by receiving rewards or incentives for achieving therapeutic goals.[2] Although such a formal process is not needed for most individuals, it may be suggested in situations where other methods have been tried and failed. Alternatively, a less formal, verbal contract can be entered into with a noncompliant patient whereby the pharmacist asks the patient to try to adhere to his or her therapy for a particular period.

    Another form of behavioral modification involves the use of patient support groups. Particularly in the case of long-term treatment and under conditions requiring significant life-style changes, support groups and on-going counseling can help the patient to self-regulate and to deal with issues that interfere with compliance as they occur.

    Behavioral modification techniques such as these may be helpful in regard to treatment for diabetes, weight loss, cholesterol control, and smoking cessation.[15]

7. *Controlled Therapy:* Controlled-therapy programs can also help noncompliant patients, particularly when long-term therapy is involved or when the patient has been dependent on caregivers administering medication previously. Such programs are sometimes organized as part of a hospital discharge program, whereby patients begin taking

responsibility for administering their own medications before discharge. This allows time for difficulties with the medication or regimen to be detected and resolved before discharge. It also trains patients to organize their medications and to remember to take them.

8. *Self-Monitoring Programs:* Patients may be assisted in self-monitoring programs that assist patients to monitor and adjust medications as needed e.g., use of a blood glucose monitor. This has also been successful in pain management, where patients can actually administer doses of analgesics at their own rates (subject to some limits). This tends to reduce the underuse or overuse of such medications and results in improved relief of symptoms.

Once again, interventions used should be tailored to the patient's needs, and multiple strategies should be employed for maximum effectiveness.[31]

Table 4.2   Methods for Resolving Noncompliance

Motivational Methods

Explain benefits of medication use

Raise patient's awareness of body cues in dictating need for medication

Explain how patient can self-evaluate

Help patient develop coping mechanisms

Tools and Techniques

Compliance aids

Enlisting support of the spouse or other family members

Increase supervision

Social-service intervention

Switching to an alternative dosing schedule or dosage form

Behavioral modification techniques

Controlled therapy

Self-monitoring programs

Follow-up to Noncompliance Intervention

Once the pharmacist has selected various techniques to resolve noncompliance, he or she should arrange and conduct follow-up visits with the patient. Having arranged with the patient when follow-up would occur, the pharmacist can either telephone the patient or speak with him in the pharmacy to determine if compliance is improved and if the planned outcomes are occurring.

Special Programs

Although compliance is largely an individual matter, groups of individuals with similar characteristics, such as age or type of condition, have similar compliance problems and therefore can be targeted with special programs to deal with noncompliance.

For example, parents of children with acute otitis media were found to have high motivation to treat the condition initially because of accuracy of the diagnosis and their children's symptoms of pain and discomfort. However, after 5 to 6 days of a 10-day antibiotic regimen, compliance decreased to only 20% to 30% because the motivation has been significantly reduced as the symptoms abated. Compliance programs for this group should therefore be aimed at increasing motivation to treat during the latter term of the treatment.[32]

The chronically ill older patient presents another situation regarding compliance intervention. The complexities of disease may lead to questions regarding accurate diagnosis and treatment; cognitive impairment may limit the ability of the patient to self-administer medications; drug reactions may be more likely; cost may be of concern; and elderly patients may be more likely than younger groups to prefer certain types of treatment over others. It has therefore been suggested that specific education programs developed for the elderly should be aimed at increased supervision of medication use as well as greater discussion with the patient to explore values and cognitive ability.[32]

Other groups of patients who have been found to benefit from special compliance programs include schizophrenic patients, sight-impaired and hearing-impaired patients, children, and the elderly.[24,27,33,34] These programs will be discussed further in Chapter 6.

Discussion of a Specific Counseling Situation

Dealing with a Noncompliant Patient: The Need for Careful Probing

An important part of refill counseling involves the identification and resolution of noncompliance. In order to do this effectively, the pharmacist must use careful probing.

Situation

Mrs. Preston is a middle-aged woman who is picking up a refill prescription for hydrochlorothiazide 50 mg. When the pharmacist checked the patient profile, she noticed that the interval since the last refill was appropriate. She proceeds to counsel the patient as follows:

<u>Pharmacist</u>: Hello, Mrs. Preston, your prescription is ready. It looks like things are going OK for you. Have you been feeling all right?
<u>Patient</u>: Yes, pretty good, but a little tired.

Pharmacist: That sounds like low potassium. You were told to drink orange juice or eat a banana every day. You are doing that aren't you?
Patient: *(feeling too foolish to admit forgetting about that)* Oh, well, sometimes.
Pharmacist: Well, try to remember in the future. I guess we'll see you in another 3 months when these run out.
Patient: OK.

Discussion

This pharmacist did not plan to investigate noncompliance with the patient because the patient profile did not indicate a problem. She made a poor attempt to assess the effectiveness of the medication and to rule out any medication-related problems. When a problem did come to light she did not pursue appropriate questioning to identify the problem or attempt to resolve it in an effective manner.

Alternate Situation

Pharmacist: Hello, Mrs. Preston, how are you today?
Patient: Oh, pretty good, but a little tired.
Pharmacist: Oh, I know the feeling. Why don't you come and have a seat over here where we can spend a few minutes discussing your medication to make sure you're getting the most benefit from it.
Patient: Thanks, that would be good.
Pharmacist: You're getting a refill of your hydrochlorothiazide. I see you've been taking it for a while now. How is it working for you?
Patient: Well, I guess it's working OK. It sure makes me lose water like it's supposed to. I even have to get up in the night to go to the bathroom. It's wearing me out.
Pharmacist: Yes, you mentioned that you've been tired. That can't be very pleasant having your sleep disturbed.
Patient: I get so tired. Sometimes I stop taking it for a few days just so I can get some rest. I know I have to keep taking it to keep my blood pressure down, so I only stop for a few days, then I start again.
Pharmacist: I see. How often would you say you stop taking them like that?
Patient: Oh, maybe every few weeks. Then my ankles get so swelled up that I take a few extra to make up for it.
Pharmacist: That doesn't sound so good. So, the problems are that you feel tired and that you have to get up during the night to go the bathroom.
Patient: Yes.
Pharmacist: Let's see what we can do about that. Can you tell me when you usually take your pills?
Patient: Well, I usually take them in the morning.
Pharmacist: Most people forget to take their pills sometimes. How often do you find you forget?

Patient: Well, several times a week I forget to take them in the morning, then I take them when I remember, usually after supper.

Pharmacist: It's important to take this medication regularly. When you stop taking them, the fluid builds up as you've found, and when you start the pills again, you have to go to the bathroom more than usual. Also, taking them late in the day increases the chance of having to get up during the night to go to the bathroom. Try taking them every day, first thing in the morning. I'll give you a calendar and a pill-reminder box to help you keep on track.

Patient: Oh, I get it now. I really need to take them regularly. Those reminders sound like a good idea to help me remember too.

Pharmacist: Now, about your tiredness. It may be a result of having to get up during the night, or it could be caused by low potassium resulting from the hydrochlorothiazide. I mentioned a while ago that with these pills you need to have a banana or a glass of orange juice every day for extra potassium. I know it's hard to remember everything. I wonder if you've been getting enough of those foods?

Patient: Oh, I forgot about that. I haven't been doing that at all.

Pharmacist: Well, that may be the problem then. I suggest that you see your doctor. I'll call to tell her about how you've been feeling, and I'll tell her that you haven't been taking the orange juice or bananas. She'll probably want to check your potassium. If it's low, she may prescribe some potassium pills to make it up.

Patient: OK. I'll make an appointment today.

Pharmacist: Do you have any questions?

Patient: No, I think I understand now that I should take the pills every day, and that if I take them in the morning, I should be OK by bedtime. And I'd better start eating those foods with potassium.

Pharmacist: Good. I'll call you in a few days to see how you're doing and to find out what the doctor suggested.

Patient: OK. I'll talk to you then. Goodbye.

Pharmacist: *returns to the dispensary to telephone the physician, then documents the intervention and discussion on the patient's profile.*

Further Discussion

This time, the pharmacist conducted a complete refill counseling session. She asked appropriate probing questions to identify noncompliance, including the details of noncompliance and factors contributing to the noncompliance. She made sure not to judge the patient's forgetfulness or lack of understanding about her medication, and made it easy for the patient to fully disclose her noncompliance. Along with the patient, the pharmacist discovered how best to resolve the noncompliance, then obtained the patient's implicit agreement to discuss it with her physician. Finally, the pharmacist arranged to follow-up with the patient to monitor the success of the resolution of noncompliance, then documented her intervention. Counseling for refill prescriptions will be further discussed in Chapter 5.

Summary

The discussion of noncompliance in this chapter has emphasized the need for the pharmacist to deal with the patient in a helping manner. The importance of keeping an open mind when dealing with noncompliant patients and of remaining nonjudgmental have also been stressed. It has been pointed out that the content and quality of communication between the patient and the pharmacist is crucial in preventing, identifying, and resolving noncompliance problems. In addition, the pharmacist should communicate in an appropriate and timely manner with physicians and other health-care workers in dealing with noncompliance by their patients. A variety of methods and tools have been discussed as they pertain to compliance counseling, and the scenario has illustrated these points.

The following three chapters will discuss more specifically the content of communication with the patient, patient–education methods and communication skills for patient counseling.

References

1. Sackett D, Snow J. The magnitude of compliance and noncompliance. In: Compliance in health care. Haynes R, Taylor D, Sakett D, eds. Baltimore: Johns Hopkins University Press. 1979:11-22.
2. Bond W, Hussar D. Detection methods and strategies for improving medication compliance. Am J Hosp Pharm. 1991;48(9):1978-1988.
3. Anon. Schering Report XIV. Kentucky Pharm. 1992;6:176-178.
4. Clepper I. Noncompliance: The invisible epidemic. Drug Topics. 1992;136(16):44-50,56-65.
5. Strand LM, Cipolle RJ, Morley PC. Pharmaceutical care: an introduction. Current Concepts, 1992. Kalamazoo, MI: The Upjohn Co. 1992:15.
6. Lasagna L. Noncompliance data and clinical outcomes: Impact on health care. Drug Topics. 1992;Supp 136(13):33-35.
7. Rudd P. Partial compliance in the treatment of hypertension: Issues and strategies. Drug Topics. 1992;Supp. 136(13):16-21.
8. Becker MH, Rosenstock IM. Compliance with medical advice. In: Health Care and Human Behavior. Steptoe A, Mathews A, eds. London: Academic Press. 1984.
9. Conrad P. The meaning of medication: Another look at compliance. Soc Sci Med. 1985; 20(1):29-37.
10. Morehead EA, Morehead L., eds. The New American Webster dictionary. Chicago: New American Library. Time Mirror, 1972.
11. Christensen D. Understanding patient drug-taking compliance. J Soc Admin Pharm. 1985; 3(2):70-77.

12. McKenney J. The clinical pharmacy and compliance. In: Compliance in health care. Haynes R, Taylor D, Sackett D, eds. Baltimore: Johns Hopkins University Press.1979:260-277.

13. Di Matteo M, DiNicola D. The compliance problem: An introduction. In: Achieving Patient Compliance. New York: Pergamon Press. 1982: 18-27.

14. Ley P. Memory for medical information. In: Communicating with Patients: Improving Communication, Satisfaction and Compliance. New York: Croom, Helm. 1988:27-52.

15. Fisher R. Patient education and compliance: A pharmacist's perspective. Pat Educ Couns. 1992;19:261-271.

16. Cockburn J, Gibberd R, Reid A, et al. Determinants of noncompliance with short term antibiotic regimens. Br Med J. 1987;295:814-818.

17. Hamilton R, Briceland L. Use of prescription-refill records to assess patient compliance. Am J Hosp Pharm. 1992;49(7):1691-1696.

18. Morris LA. A survey of patients' receipt of prescription drug information. Med Care. 1982;20(6):596-605.

19. Slovic P, Kraus N, Lappe H, et al. Risk perception of prescription drugs: Report on a survey in Canada. Pharm Pract. 1992;8(1):30-37.

20. Nichol M, McCombs J, Johnson K, et al. The effects of consultation on over-the-counter medication purchasing decisions. Med Care. 1992;30(11):989-1003.

21. Regner MJ, et al. Effectiveness of a printed leaflet for enabling patients to use digoxin side effect information. Drug Intell Clin Pharm. 1987;21(2):200-204.

22. Seltzer A, et al. Effect of patient education on medication compliance. Can J Psych. 1980;25(12): 638-645.

23. McBean BJ, Blackburn JL. An evaluation of four methods of pharmacist-conducted patient education. Can Pharm J. 1982;115(5):167-172.

24. Morris LA, et. al. A survey of the effects of oral contraceptive patient information. JAMA;238(23):2504-2508.

25. Simpkins C, Wenzloff N. Evaluation of a computer reminder system in the enhancement of patient medication refill compliance. Drug Intell Clin Pharm. 1986;20(10):799-802.

26. Nagle BA, German TC, Coons SJ, et al. Developing a compliance screening program to monitor and minimize noncompliance in the elderly. Abstract of Meeting Presentation. ASHP Midyear Clinical Meeting 26 P-456D, Dec. 1991.

27. Opdycke RA, Ascione F, Shimp L, et al. A systematic approach to educating elderly patients about their medications. Pat Educ Couns. 1992;19:43-60.

28. Stoudemire A, Thompson T. Medication noncompliance: Systematic approaches to evaluation and intervention. Gen Hosp Psych. 1983; 5(12): 233-239.

29. Eisenberg S, Delaney DJ. Working with reluctant clients. In: The Counseling Process. 2nd ed. Chicago: Rand McNally, 1977.

30. Leventhal H, Safer, MA, Panagis DM. The impact of communication on the self-regulation of health beliefs, decisions, and behavior. Health Educ Q. 1983;10(1):3-29.

31. Given C, Given B, Coyle B. The effect of patient characteristics and beliefs on responses to behavioral intervention for control of chronic disease. Pat Educ Couns. 1984;6(3):137-140.

32. Owens N. Patient noncompliance: Subset analysis. Drug Topics. 1992;Supp 136(13):11-15.

33. Moore SR. Cognitive variants in the elderly: Integral part of medication counseling. Drug Intell Clin Pharm. 1983;17(11):840-842

34. Schoepp G. For kids only. Drug Merch. 1990;71(1):26-31.

5
MEDICATION-COUNSELING BASICS

Having considered the goals of counseling, and patients' needs and concerns with respect to medication use, let us now turn to the specifics of the counseling session. The patient–pharmacist encounter consists of an exchange of information, feelings, beliefs, values, and ideas between the patient and the pharmacist—much like any other conversation between two people. It *should not* consist of a one-sided lecture by the pharmacist.

The specific information exchanged during that encounter will depend on the nature of the encounter and the reason why the encounter is taking place. The patient–pharmacist encounter may involve a new patient or a returning patient. It may concern a new medication or a refill, a prescription or a nonprescription medication. The encounter may also involve a medication-history interview, a medication monitoring interview, or a response by the pharmacist to an inquiry by the patient regarding a specific condition, symptom, or medication.

It may be useful at this point to refer back to Chapter 2 and review the goals of the counseling process, remembering that there are both counseling and educational goals. The pharmacist's main purpose is to help patients maximize the benefits they will gain from their medication. This involves enhancing patients' skills, knowledge, attitudes, and behavior with respect to their illnesses and their medications.

Patient counseling is an integral part of the provision of pharmaceutical care as many of the steps in the pharmaceutical care process involve pharmacist–patient interaction through patient counseling. As such, the following discussion of medication counseling will refer to the pharmaceutical care process as they apply.

OBRA-'90 requires only that an "offer" be made to counsel for "new" prescriptions, and it does not articulate whether this should be done by the pharmacist or a delegated individual. However, the National Association of Boards of Pharmacy (NABP) advocates that the offer be made personally to each patient (not via a posted sign); that the pharmacist should offer counseling for all prescriptions, new or refill; and that the pharmacist should not delegate the counseling responsibilities.[1]

Preparing for the Counseling Encounter

In the case of prescription counseling for a return patient, the pharmacist has an opportunity to prepare for the encounter during the dispensing process. Through review of the patient's medication record, the pharmacist may identify real or potential problems such as noncompliance (over or under use), drug interactions, allergies to prescribed drugs, or interference with existing conditions. In addition, the pharmacist should note any information that may affect counseling or medication use such as disabilities (e.g., impaired hearing or eyesight) or language barriers. In the case of a new patient to the pharmacy, this information needs to be gathered through a medication-history interview, which is discussed in detail later in this chapter.

Once real or potential problems are identified either from the medication record or history, appropriate prevention or resolution of problems can be considered and appropriate action can be taken. This may involve discussion with the physician, consultation of references, and/or consideration of the compliance resolution methods described earlier. Further problem identification and resolution will be carried out during the patient counseling encounter.

Preparation for the patient-counseling encounter may also involve a review by the pharmacist of information concerning the medication and the condition being treated. In addition, any available print information regarding the condition being treated and the medication should be selected for the patient.

A further consideration the pharmacist should make before entering into discussion with the patient is the need for privacy. All counseling should be conducted with a relative degree of privacy in order to encourage the patient to disclose appropriate personal information, as well as to allow the pharmacist to interact with the patient in an atmosphere free from distractions. If the medication involves a condition that might be embarrassing for the patient, instructions that may be complicated, or issues that need to be addressed that may be time consuming, counseling will be more suitable – and more productive – if it takes place in a private area. If this is not possible, it may be better to suggest to the patient that the counseling be carried out over the telephone. The issue of privacy will be discussed further in Chapter 9.

The Counseling Process

In general, the counseling process should proceed as illustrated in the flow chart in Figure 5.1. This figure suggests five phases: **1)** the opening discussion; **2)** discussion to gather information and identify problems; **3)** discussion to prevent and resolve problems and provide appropriate information; **4)** the closing discussion; and **5)** follow-up discussions.

The manner adopted in asking questions and the wording used to present information may be critical to the outcome of the counseling encounter. Suggested dialogues to use during the counseling encounter are provided in Appendix B, and the communication skills involved are discussed in Chapter 7.

The need to introduce the counseling is especially important if the patient has never before been counseled by a pharmacist. In such circumstances, patients are sometimes disconcerted by the pharmacist's attention, unprepared to discuss personal information, and possibly unwilling to spend the necessary time talking with the pharmacist. Take for example the following counseling situation:

Counseling Situation

Mrs. Hampton is a middle aged woman. It is her first time in this particular pharmacy, and she has not previously been counseled by a pharmacist. She gives the pharmacist a new prescription for tetracycline. The pharmacist notices that Mrs. Hampton's name is not familiar.

Figure 5.1   Flow Chart For Patient Counseling

Opening Discussion

- Introduction   • Explain purpose of counseling

Discussion to Gather Information and Identify Problems

New Patient
- Gather patient information
- Conduct medication history

Returning Patient
- Confirm patient information
- Confirm medication-history information

What is the purpose of counseling?

New Rx
- Patient's present knowledge about medication and condition?
- Potential problems

Refill Rx / Monitoring
- Compliance problems?
- Evidence of side effects?
- Effectiveness of treatment
- Potential problems

Nonprescription Drugs
- Description and duration of symptoms
- Has physician been consulted previously?
- What treatment has been used previously?

Identify Problems and Educational Needs

Discussion to Prevent or Resolve Problems and Educate

New or Refill Rx / Monitoring
- Discuss real or potential problems
- Agree on alternatives
- Implement plan
- Discuss outcomes and monitoring
- Provide information as necessary

Nonprescription Drugs

Medication Recommended
- Name
- Purpose
- Directions
- Side effects
- Precautions
- Future treatment
- Reassurance

No Medication Recommended
- Advise patient to see physician
- Suggest nondrug treatment
- Provide information as necessary
- Reassurance

Closing Discussion

- Recap   • Get feedback   • Encourage questions

Follow-up Discussions

Pharmacist: Hello, Mrs. Hampton. Have you had prescriptions filled here before?

Patient: No, I usually go to the pharmacy close to my office.

Pharmacist: You'll have to fill out this patient history form then. What's your address, phone number, and drug-plan information?

Patient: *(indignantly)* If this is going to be a problem, I can go back to the other pharmacy.

Pharmacist: *(quickly)* No, no. We can fill the prescription for you here. Just fill this form out while you're waiting. I just need your name, address, and drug-plan information to get started.

Patient: *(reluctantly)* OK.

...10 minutes pass

Pharmacist: Mrs. Hampton. Your prescription is ready now.

Patient: *(returns to the pharmacy counter and hands over the patient history form)* Here's your form. I don't know why you need all this information. My doctor has it all.

Pharmacist: It's just for our records. Now, let me see. *(glances at the patient history form)* You seem to have filled this in correctly. You didn't list any nonprescription medications. What about those?

Patient: *(getting more aggravated by the minute, not realizing that the antacid she takes occasionally for stomach upset and the calcium supplement she takes are considered nonprescription medications)* I don't see the point in all this information, just let me have my prescription.

Pharmacist: *(not wanting to aggravate the patient any further)* Well, I guess that's OK then. I'll just take a minute to go over your new medication with you.

Patient: Look, the doctor told me all about how to take it four times daily for 10 days, on an empty stomach. Now, can I go?

Pharmacist: Yes. Well, here's some more information on this sheet. *(attempts to review it with the patient)*

Patient: *(snatches the sheet from the pharmacist's hands)* Fine, I'll read it at home.

Pharmacist: OK. Well, if you have any questions after you read this feel free to call.

Patient: Sure. *(walks away thinking)* What a waste of time! Next time I'll just go back to the other pharmacy. They never hassle me like this. *(when she gets home she takes the prescription out of the bag and throws the bag with the information sheet inside into the garbage, forgetting that it is there)*

Discussion

This pharmacist obviously had very good intentions to attempt to learn the patient's medication history before proceeding to counsel this new patient. But something went wrong! The patient wasn't at all receptive. In fact, she viewed the discussion as an aggravation. As a result, the pharmacist was not able to develop sufficient rapport with the patient to allow complete assessment of the medication history, or even to conduct appropriate counseling for a new prescription. If the pharmacist had properly conducted an opening discussion and inquired about the necessary information appropriately, the situation might have ended differently. The pharmacist would have discovered the potential drug interactions and would have been able to proceed to counsel the patient.

The Opening Discussion

The purpose of the opening discussion is to develop a helping relationship with the patient and a sense of trust in the pharmacist. This is an important step in the pharmaceutical care process as it may strongly influence the ability of the pharmacist to gather information and to make appropriate decisions regarding the nature of the patient's real or potential problems and methods to resolve them.

The pharmacist should attempt to set a personal and conversational tone. If the patient and pharmacist have not previously met, the pharmacist should introduce himself, stating his name and position clearly. The patient's identity should also be verified to ensure that the correct patient is receiving the prescription and to confirm that the person picking up the prescription is indeed the patient. The patient's name should then be used during the counseling session to help personalize the encounter.

If a third party is picking up the medication, the pharmacist must determine whether the information can be reliably transmitted to the patient through the third party. If at all possible, it is advisable to arrange to speak with the patient in person or by telephone to at least confirm that all information and instructions have been relayed and understood, and to explore any problems or concerns that the patient may have. OBRA-'90 requires an "offer" to counsel the patient be made "in person" whenever possible, or through access to toll-free telephone service.[1]

If possible, this initial phase of patient counseling should occur when the patient is placing the medication request. Although a clerk or pharmacy technician often receives the order, the pharmacist can secure a better relationship with the patient and can anticipate future problems during this initial encounter with the patient. For example, the patient may hand over the prescription and say, "I guess I'd better get this prescription filled now, although I really don't see any point in it." Unless the clerk or technician taking the prescription relayed this comment, the pharmacist would have missed an opportunity to explore the patient's concerns.

As a further attempt to set the patient at ease and create a friendly atmosphere, the pharmacist should try to engage the patient in casual conversation. For example, the pharmacist might comment on the weather or inquire after the patient's family. Although this "warm-up" should be brief, it should not appear rushed.

Following the introduction and warm-up, the purpose of the counseling should be made clear to the patient. The pharmacist should explain what will follow, why, and how long it will take. This will prepare the patient for the potentially personal nature of the discussion and may motivate the patient to participate.

If the patient indicates that he or she does not have time to discuss the medication immediately (even after being told of the importance of the information to the outcome of the therapy), then it may be necessary to arrange for the conversation to take place, either in person or by telephone, at an alternate time. OBRA-'90 does not require the pharmacist to provide consultation services if the patient refuses, but it does recommend that pharmacists make an effort to convince the patient that this is a desirable exercise. However, as noted earlier, it can be very difficult to counsel an unwilling patient, and beyond a certain point, any attempt to do so is likely to prove a waste of time and effort. In this case, the pharmacist should be sure to document that the offer to counsel was made and that the patient refused.

Discussion to Gather Information and Identify Problems

In this phase of the counseling encounter, the pharmacist's aim is to gather any information from the patient with a view to identifying real or potential problems with the medication, as well as to identify the patient's information needs. The content of this discussion will vary depending on whether it involves a new patient or a patient returning to the same pharmacy and on whether it concerns a nonprescription drug, a new prescription, or a refill prescription. A medication-monitoring interview would proceed in a similar manner for a refill prescription. Nonprescription drug counseling will be discussed later in this chapter.

Discussion with a New Patient

If the patient is new to the pharmacy, the pharmacist will need to gather basic patient information. OBRA-'90 requires Medicaid pharmacy providers to "make a reasonable effort to obtain, record, and maintain the following information: name, address, telephone number, age and gender."[1] In addition, OBRA-'90 requires that information be recorded regarding the patient's history where significant, including disease state or states, known allergies and drug reactions, and a comprehensive list of medications and relevant devices. The pharmacist's comments relevant to the individual's drug therapy must also be noted.[1]

The gathering of the patient's history through a medication-history interview will be discussed in further detail later in this chapter. It will be explained that this interview should elucidate more than the above facts. It may therefore be more practical simply to gather the above information and brief details pertinent to the medication being dispensed during the medication-counseling session, and to schedule a complete medication interview for a time more convenient for the pharmacist and patient.

Discussion With a Returning Patient

For a returning patient, certain information should already be available from a previously conducted medication history and from the patient record or chart. In this case, the pharmacist simply has to inquire to confirm that there are no changes such as new conditions or medications received elsewhere, either prescription or nonprescription.

Discussion for a New Prescription

If the encounter involves a new prescription, the following information should be obtained from the patient, in addition to the patient information and medication-history information discussed:

1. *Previous Use:* The pharmacist must first determine whether the patient has ever taken the medication before. Even for a returning patient for whom the medication does not appear on the patient record, the patient may have received the medication from another pharmacy, directly from the physician, or during a hospital visit. If the patient has taken the medication previously, the remainder of the counseling will be geared to a refill, rather than a new prescription.

2. *Purpose for Medication:* If the prescription is indeed new, the pharmacist must determine the condition being treated and the patient's under-standing and perception of this. The pharmacist should ask what the physician has told the patient about the purpose of the medication. This will allow the pharmacist to gauge the level of the patient's understand-ing about his or her condition and the purpose of the medication, and will allow the patient the opportunity to express concerns or problems regarding his or her condition. The pharmacist will then be able to assess the patient's information needs in this regard, and to identify potential misunderstanding or lack of motivation that may lead to noncompliance.

   This discussion also provides the pharmacist with an indication of the patient's language level. The pharmacist should then adopt this language during the following discussion as much as possible (e.g., if the patient refers to his epileptic seizures as "blackouts," the pharmacist should use the same term). If knowledge of English is a concern, then this must be addressed (see Chapter 8 for further discussion).

   Through the discussion the pharmacist will also gain information to evaluate whether the prescribed medication is an appropriate choice. Although, the patient's view of the purpose of the medication may or may not be accurate, it will indicate gross errors. If possible, the pharmacist should supplement this information with the actual medical diagnosis or treatment goal from the physician.

3. *Medication Regimen:* The pharmacist must then determine the patient's understanding of how the medication is to be used. The pharmacist should ask the patient what the physician has said about medication use and whether the patient anticipates any problems taking the medication

as prescribed. This will allow the pharmacist to assess the patient's information needs and may save time if the patient demonstrates that he or she already understands the information clearly. Again, this will give the patient the opportunity to raise anticipated concerns or problems with the regimen, and will allow the pharmacist to identify potential noncompliance or dosing problems.

4. *Treatment Goal:* The patient may also be asked what he or she would like to accomplish by taking this medication. This will further elucidate any perceptions regarding medication use that would lead to problems.

Discussion for a Refill Prescription and Medication-Monitoring Interview

If the encounter involves a refill prescription or a medication-monitoring interview, the following information should be gathered, in addition to the patient information and medication-history information discussed above, where necessary:

1. *Details of Medication Use:* The pharmacist should determine how the patient is using the medication and whether the patient has experienced any difficulty thus far in taking the medication (e.g., overuse or underuse). If a review of the patient record has indicated noncompliance, questioning should follow concerning the actual frequency of medication use and the possible reasons for noncompliance. As stressed in the previous chapter, this should be a gentle probing, not an inquisition. Factors contributing to noncompliance should be explored as discussed in the previous chapter (e.g., difficulties with dosing regimen, misunderstanding about use, perceptions about need, etc.).

2. *Effectiveness of Medication:* The pharmacist should also determine whether the medication is effective. The pharmacist should ask if the medication is helping and if it is accomplishing what was expected. In addition to the patient's perceptions, the pharmacist should ask specific questions about symptoms that would indicate medication effectiveness in a clinical sense (e.g., blood pressure levels). The patient may not be the most accurate source of this information so that, where possible, this should be supplemented with actual clinical data from the physician or patient chart.

    This discussion also allows the pharmacist to identify any misgivings or concerns that the patient might have (e.g., the patient may report that his blood pressure readings have been reduced but that he or she doesn't notice any difference in how he or she feels, and therefore sees little point in continuing).

3. *Presence of Adverse Effects:* The pharmacist should also determine if any adverse effects are occurring. He or she should ask whether the patient has felt any different than usual while on this medication. Such questioning should always be balanced by a general statement about the rarity of adverse effects, and about the necessity of checking for signs

to allow for prompt treatment should they occur. Probing regarding specific adverse effects can follow. Note that in this discussion, symptoms should be described rather than the medical names of conditions (e.g., "discolored tongue" rather than "black hairy tongue"). It is important to gather information regarding the duration and severity of side effects in order to allow the pharmacist and physician to decide if a change in medication is warranted or if the side effects are manageable. The patient's perceptions and quality of life are important here since he may be unwilling to tolerate a side effect that is considered clinically manageable (e.g., constipation).

Discussion to Prevent or Resolve Problems and Educate

Now that any real or potential problems have been identified, a plan can be developed to deal with problems where necessary and to monitor progress. In addition, information needs that have been identified should now be satisfied.

Developing a Pharmaceutical Care Plan During the Patient Counseling Process

Having gathered complete information, the pharmacist is now in a position to develop a pharmaceutical care plan.[2] This will require some thought on the pharmacist's part, as well as some discussion with the patient. If real or potential problems have been identified, then the pharmacist should inform the patient that there appears to be some important things to discuss and negotiate with the patient in the order of importance.[2]

Next, desired pharmacotherapeutic outcomes for each real or potential problem should be established.[2] This should be done through discussion with the patient, and should include ways the patient could identify these outcomes.[2] For example, for a patient experiencing constipation as a result of medication use, the pharmacist may discuss the situation with the patient and may determine that the patient would like the constipation alleviated so that his normal once daily bowel movement would return, and that this would occur by the end of 2 weeks.

If discussion with the patient resulted in a conclusion that the patient's therapy should be altered, then the pharmacist must identify alternatives.[2] These alternatives should be discussed with the patient, and if a change in a prescribed drug is involved, then with the physician. For example, the patient experiencing constipation as a result of medication use may require a change to a medication that does not cause constipation, or the addition of an extra medication to alleviate constipation.

As a result of these deliberations, the pharmacist should then determine the best pharmacotherapeutic solution and individualize the therapeutic regimen.[2] The patient should again be involved in a discussion regarding the choice of drug, dose, formulation, and regimen. For example, for the patient with constipation, the choice of laxative should be discussed with the patient to be sure that it meets his or her wishes as far as dosage form, time to effect, and frequency of need.

Once this is decided, the pharmacist should discuss a drug-monitoring plan with the patient.[2] This may involve a telephone call to the patient, who would keep track of symptoms; the patient returning to the physician at set intervals; or the patient returning to the pharmacy at set intervals.

Finally, any changes in therapy and a plan for monitoring therapy should then be initiated and documented by the pharmacist.[2]

Providing Information

The pharmacist needs to provide the patient with information about the medication he or she is receiving and, if necessary, about the condition for which he or she is being treated. As discussed in Chapter 4, this may prevent any potential compliance problems (provided it is presented in an appropriate way).

In the past, there has been some controversy about how much information a patient should be given about his or her medication and condition, and about which health professional should provide it. As mentioned in Chapter 1, pharmacists may be found liable if they fail to provide sufficient information. Standards of practice now require pharmacists to provide at least minimal information to patients about their medications. This is required by law for Medicaid patients and in many states, for all patients.[1]

Although legislation and regulations in some jurisdictions clearly specify the details to be provided, the pharmacist must often decide the extent of detail that is appropriate on the basis of several considerations. One consideration is that of the patient's rights. Over the past few years, members of the public have become increasingly aware of their rights to know about their drug treatments, alternative treatments, and possible risks of treatment.[3] Another consideration is the pharmacist's perception of the patient's ability to understand the information based on the patient's level of education, language barriers, and so on. There are also concerns about infringing on the physician's responsibility. The pharmacist must weigh these considerations for each individual patient and situation.

Reference sources designed to assist the pharmacist in the provision of medication information to patients are listed in Appendix A. Additional information sources, such as print information and audiovisual materials, may be given to the patient for future reference either at this stage of the counseling session or later during the closing phase of the session. Patient information materials will be discussed in Chapter 6 and in Appendix A.

The type of information that should be provided by the pharmacist will vary with nonprescription drugs, new prescriptions, and refill prescriptions. Nonprescription drug counseling will be discussed later in the chapter. Information that the patient indicated knowledge of during the previous phase of counseling, can be omitted. In addition, the patient may have asked specific questions about his therapy or condition which need to be addressed here.

Refill Prescription and Drug-Monitoring Interview: If problems such as noncompliance, side effects, or adverse effects were not detected during the information-gathering phase, the patient may not need to be given any new information. In this case, the pharmacist might simply reinforce previous information provided to the patient about precautions that should be observed while on the medication, about the need to continue with the medication, and about the availability of refills.

Resolution of compliance problems may involve providing information about the patient's medical condition; information about the way the medication is intended to work; reassurance about the efficacy of the medication; suggestions for altering the regimen to improve compliance; or suggestions for further discussion with the physician.

If side effects or adverse effects were detected, information needed from the pharmacist may include actions to reduce side effects (e.g., take with food); reassurance that the effects are mild or that they are likely to decrease with continued medication use; methods to continue monitoring side effects and actions to take if they become more severe and recommendation to consult a physician for further assessment.

New Prescription: The types of information that may be necessary to provide for a new prescription include the following:

1. *The name and description of the drug.* Although the name of the drug appears on the label of the prescription, generic and trade names may be somewhat confusing for the patient, and the relationship between the two should be clarified. The dosage form of the drug should be made clear, e.g. liquid medicine to be taken by mouth.

2. *The purpose of the medication and, briefly, how it is intended to work.* This information should be stated in the simplest terms. If necessary, more detail may be provided regarding the condition being treated.

3. *How and when to take the medication.* The patient should be shown the label on the prescription package, and the instructions should be read from it. Further explanation may be necessary in some cases, for example, that "every 4 hours" means "around the clock."

   If the medication must be ingested or applied in a particular way, the patient should be instructed concerning the proper procedure, then should be encouraged to practice it. If the instructions are complicated or require skill development, as in the case of inhaler use, the patient should be asked to repeat the instructions back to the pharmacist (placebo inhalers are available from manufacturers for demonstration purposes). In addition, any special directions or precautions regarding preparation or use should be provided (e.g., use in a ventilated area; may stain clothes).

4. *Compliance suggestions and techniques for self-monitoring.* The patient should be asked if he or she foresees any difficulty in using the medication as instructed, and if so, suggestions for overcoming them should be made, as discussed in the previous chapter.

   Potential noncompliance problems should also be anticipated as a result of previous information gathered, and suggestions should be made to prevent noncompliance such as techniques to remember medication use, suggestions of how to involve family or friends, etc.

Information should also be provided about what to do if a dose is missed, particularly if a missed dose would be critical (e.g., with oral contraceptives).

Techniques for self-monitoring drug therapy are also important in preventing noncompliance. This may involve suggesting the patient learn to take his or her own blood pressure readings or keep a diary of symptom severity and improvement.

5. *Side effects and adverse effects.* As noted above, the depth to which information on this subject is provided will depend on the patient and the situation. The pharmacist should preface the discussion with a statement about the rarity of such effects. As discussed in Chapter 3, when patients are properly prepared, they are likely to feel more in control of the situation and are less apprehensive about their medication use.

Only the symptoms of adverse effects should be described, and complicated names of conditions (e.g., blood dyscrasia) should be avoided. It is very important that the patient be told how to handle the symptoms, whether by employing actions that will minimize them (such as taking the medication with food or plenty of water) or by contacting the prescribing physician immediately.

The patient should be told which symptoms are minor and of little concern and which symptoms necessitate contact with the physician. The patient should always be reassured that these effects are not likely to occur, but that, if they do, early detection and treatment are essential.

6. *Precautions and contraindications.* The patient should always be advised about any precautions associated with the medication—for example, that the medication could harm a fetus or be transmitted to an infant through the mother's breast milk.

The pharmacist should also make the patient aware of possible interactions with certain nonprescription medications and alcohol. If a number of possible interactions exist, it might be more useful to instruct the patient to consult with the pharmacist or prescribing physician before using any nonprescription medications, and to inform any future physicians or pharmacists of current medication use. The topic of alcohol use should be addressed in a nonjudgmental manner, explaining the reason for mention. Suggested wording for such discussions is provided in Appendix B.

Contraindications to medication use should also be addressed in case the patient develops the conditions in the future. For example, if a patient was to decide to try to become pregnant, a potentially teratogenic drug should be discontinued.

7. *Storage instructions*. Any special storage instructions, such as the need to refrigerate the medication, should be stated, even if the relevant information appears on an auxiliary label affixed to the package.

8. *Refill information and pharmacist monitoring plan*. The patient should be informed if the physician has indicated that the prescription may be refilled. If no such instructions have been supplied with the prescription, the patient should be asked whether the physician gave any verbal instructions regarding follow-up. If the physician has not discussed these matters with the patient, then the patient should be advised to consult with the physician. The patient also needs to know how to evaluate the effectiveness of the medication from self-monitoring and the basis on which to decide whether, or when, to discontinue medication use (e.g., what blood pressure should be and what to do if it registers above or below a given range).

Closing Discussion

In closing the patient-counseling encounter, it is important to allow the patient an opportunity to consider the information he or she has received and to ask any further questions. If the patient appears to be confused or if a language problem is suspected, it may be useful to ask the patient to repeat the most important information, such as directions for use. People are often unsure of themselves and fear that they may appear stupid if they ask questions. The pharmacist needs to reassure patients that they should feel free to ask anything at all or to discuss any concerns, whether now or later.

The closing discussion should also be used to reiterate and emphasize the most important points of the counseling, since the last message heard is usually the one that is remembered best.

Additional information sources such as written information, if available, may be provided to the patient at this point rather than during the information-giving phase of the session.

Follow-up Discussion

With the monitoring plan set in place, the pharmacist can start to follow the patient's progress and may determine the degree of success of treatment and of the plan implemented during counseling.[2] This important part of pharmaceutical care requires the pharmacist to take responsibility for ensuring that outcomes of drug therapy are positive. Refill counseling involves documenting any changes to the treatment plan and documentation regarding success of the plan to date as evidenced by the discussion with the patient.

This phase of counseling is difficult to implement when patients do not always frequent the same pharmacy. The pharmacist can help to implement follow-up for new prescriptions by explaining to the patient that this service will occur if he or she continues to patronize this pharmacy exclusively.

This is only a suggested protocol, and the patient may alter the flow at any point by asking a specific question requiring immediate discussion. If the question does not relate specifically to the medication counseling, however, the pharmacist might choose to postpone the discussion until after the counseling is completed. In any event, the question should not be ignored.

The pharmacist must also decide where to place the emphasis in the counseling protocol to maximize its effectiveness and efficiency. This involves "tailoring" the counseling to the specific patient, medication, condition, and situation. Difficult situations, such as counseling an angry patient, may also require alterations in the process. "Tailoring" counseling and dealing with difficult situations will be discussed in Chapter 8.

Nonprescription Drug Counseling

Before discussing the protocol for nonprescription drug counseling, it is useful to review the issues of self-care and self-treatment, the need for nonprescription drug counseling, and a brief history regarding the guidelines for nonprescription drug counseling by pharmacists.

Self-Care and Self-Treatment

Self-care has been defined as "a process whereby a lay person can function effectively on his or her own behalf in health promotion and decision making, in disease prevention, detection, and treatment at the level of the primary health resource in the health-care system."[4] Although self-care activities can range from breast self-examination to performing home pregnancy tests, or simply regular exercise, a frequent activity is self-treatment with medication.[5]

It has been estimated that Americans experience one potentially self-treatable health problem every 3 days.[6] Nonprescription drugs are used by many people to treat these conditions; one study found that 90% of those surveyed used nonprescription drugs, 8% of whom reported using them very often.[7] Nonprescription drugs are used either on a regular basis for chronic conditions such as stomach ulcers, or intermittently, for acute conditions such as colds.

There is a growing trend toward self-care, and consumers often view self-medication as a right.[8] Part of the trend toward self-care has been the greater availability of effective nonprescription drugs. Beginning in 1972, the FDA has been conducting a comprehensive review of over-the-counter drug products, resulting in a gradual switch of many prescription drugs to nonprescription drug status.[8,9] Some states, such as Florida, California, and Missouri, have established limited prescribing authority for the pharmacist, extending the drugs available for self-treatment beyond the traditional nonprescription items.[8]

Self-treatment by the patient has advantages for both the individual and the health-care system. To relieve minor symptoms and ailments, patients can more conveniently and more readily treat themselves than if they seek professional help. Self-treatment also relieves medical services of a heavy burden, resulting in lower costs to individuals as well as state and federal governments. Apparently nonprescription drugs account for 60% of medications purchased by Americans, but only 2% of total U.S. health care expenditures, making it a cost-effective form of health care.[5]

Other factors contributing to the self-care movement include improved education among Americans, increased health awareness and availability of health information, escalating health care costs, an aging population with more health problems, advances in the technology of diagnostic aids and monitoring devices, and the increasingly hurried lifestyle of many Americans.[5]

Need for Nonprescription Drug Counseling by Pharmacists

Nonprescription drugs are considered to be relatively safe for use without professional supervision as long as labeled directions are followed.[6] This is not necessarily the case, however, since a wide range of potential problems can arise, including interactions with other prescribed or nonprescribed medicines or alcohol; interference with existing chronic conditions; interference with the course of pregnancy or fetal development; excessive dosing or chronic use leading to physical damage and habituation or addiction; delay in receiving a correct diagnosis and treatment for more serious disease; and adverse effects or allergic reactions.[10] Many of the problems have been detected through studies of hospital admissions or patient surveys.[11-13] One study of hospital admissions found 26% of drug-related admissions over a 2-month period were due to ASA.[11] In particular, surveys with the elderly have found problems with nonprescription drugs, for example 56% of the elderly in a Florida survey were found to be using a nonprescription drug with inappropriate dose or indication.[12]

Consumers need help in making decisions regarding self-treatment. Pharmacists are in an ideal position to provide the advice needed to ensure safe and effective self-treatment, because they are often the patient's first point of contact with the health-care system.[14] It has been suggested that pharmaceutical care should not be relegated exclusively to prescription drug products.[5] The four outcomes that are sought by pharmacists in providing pharmaceutical care (curing disease, reducing or eliminating symptoms, arresting or slowing a disease process, or prevention of disease or its symptoms) can often be achieved with the use of nonprescription drugs, either at the request of the consumer or by the pharmacist's recommendation.[5]

Guidelines for Nonprescription Drug Counseling
Standards for Care

Up until the mid-1960s, pharmacists had no guidelines with respect to nonprescription drug counseling. Activities were often limited to directing the customer to the item on the shelf, answering only specific questions, suggesting that the patient ask a doctor, or selling the newest or most expensive product. In 1965, the American Pharmaceutical Association (APhA) recognized the need by pharmacists for comprehensive information and guidelines regarding nonprescription drug counseling.[15] In 1966, APhA published a series of articles on various classes of nonprescription drugs, and this provided the basis for the first "Handbook of Non-Prescription Drugs," in September, 1967.

An important part of the information provided in the "Handbook of Nonprescription Drugs," were the guidelines provided in each chapter regarding questions to ask the patient. Later editions elaborated on ways that pharmacists should assess patients who inquire about symptoms or ask for a nonprescription medication and on ways to determine the most appropriate action in each particular case.[14]

The most recent edition of the "Handbook of Nonprescription Drugs" clearly states that the course of action chosen by the pharmacist might include any one, or a combination, of the following:[14]

1. Referral to a physician for a medical opinion;
2. Recommendation of a nonprescription drug and/or nondrug treatment followed by selection of the most appropriate product and specific recommendations for its use;
3. Reassurance that no treatment is necessary.

Screening versus Diagnosing and Prescribing

When pharmacists counsel patients about nonprescription drugs, are they diagnosing and prescribing? Pharmacists generally do not have the knowledge, skills, or training required to make medical diagnoses, except in specific situations (e.g., in the case of certain products designated in Florida). They can, however, perform a triage or screening function.[14] By reviewing the symptoms and considering various other factors, the pharmacist can differentiate between symptoms indicative of a serious condition that requires formal medical referral and symptoms that indicate self-limiting conditions amenable to symptomatic treatment. The pharmacist can decide when to refer, when to suggest no treatment, and when to suggest self-medication. This is the essence of screening—the sorting out and classification of patients presenting in the pharmacy with various conditions, to determine priority of need and proper place and type of treatment.

The Nonprescription-Drug-Counseling Process

As discussed previously, the manner of questioning and of presenting information to the patient can be critical to the outcome of the counseling encounter. Suggested dialogue for the nonprescription-drug-counseling process is provided in Appendix B. As illustrated in Figure 5.1, nonprescription drug counseling should proceed through the same five stages that characterize prescription drug counseling, although the content differs somewhat.

Opening Discussion

As in prescription drug counseling, the purpose of the opening phase is to establish a helping relationship with patients and to help them to feel comfortable discussing their symptoms and health concerns. The nonprescription counseling encounter may begin in a number of ways—with the patient approaching the pharmacist to ask for a recommendation with regard to a particular condition; with the patient asking for a particular product; or with the pharmacist approaching the patient to offer help in selecting a product.

Although patients' requests for help are often handled by a pharmacy technician or clerk, any such questions should be referred to the pharmacist. The atmosphere of the pharmacy and the availability of the pharmacist are important to encourage patients to come forward with requests regarding self-care. In one study, only 34% of people felt that the pharmacist was easy to approach, and in another, only 40% said they had sought the pharmacist's advice during the last year.[16,17] Ways to improve atmosphere and availability will be discussed in Chapter 9.

Pharmacists should not wait for patients to make requests, but should be pro-active and offer their services to patients selecting a nonprescription drug. Patients often do not ask the pharmacist for advice about nonprescription drugs because they believe that they know all that is necessary or because they are unaware of potential problems.

Since patients often do not expect to be counseled about a nonprescription medication, it is important to introduce the purpose of the questioning that will follow in the next phase. The pharmacist should explain to the patient the need for further questioning in a way that does not judge or belittle (e.g., "I'll need to ask you a few questions to find out the best medication for your situation," rather than, "I'd better ask you some questions to make sure you're buying the right thing").

As with prescription counseling, it is necessary to consider the personal and potentially embarrassing nature of the discussion and to provide at least a degree of privacy.

Discussion to Gather Information and Identify Problems

Since part of the aim of nonprescription drug counseling is to screen for appropriate self-treatment, the information-gathering phase is more extensive here than it is in prescription drug counseling.

The following information should be gathered:

1. *Identity of the patient.* In many cases, the customer may be purchasing a nonprescription medication for another person. If the customer is familiar with the patient's medical history and symptoms, it may be possible to proceed with counseling. If not, however, it may be necessary to contact the patient later, either by telephone or in person.

2. *Description of the patient.* The approximate age of the patient should be determined, because special considerations are likely to be involved with the very young or the very old. Elderly people and infants under 2 years of age often present with symptoms differently or react to medications differently than do other members of the population.

Women of child-bearing age should always be asked if they are pregnant or breast feeding before medication is recommended.

3. *Medical history.* Conditions such as high blood pressure, diabetes, heart disease, or liver or kidney disease are often contraindications to nonprescription drug use. Similarly, the patient may be allergic to certain ingredients in nonprescription drugs. Indeed, the symptoms that the patient intends to self-treat may be associated in some way with such conditions. The pharmacist must assess these possible relationships and any contraindications that might be present.

4. *Other medication used.* Many medications may potentially interact with nonprescription drugs. Also, certain symptoms presented for self-treatment—such as rashes, difficulty breathing or urinating, or upset stomach—may be side effects or adverse effects of medication.

5. *Previous diagnosis and/or treatment of the symptoms.* This information will help the pharmacist to determine the products that are most suitable at this point. Patients sometimes want confirmation of their physician's diagnosis, or they disagree with it and want to self-treat even when advised against it. They may also have tried certain remedies in the past with varying degrees of success.

6. *Symptom evaluation.* Thorough questioning is necessary to determine the nature of the patient's symptoms. Patients often omit information or describe symptoms in unclear or misleading ways. Careful probing and clarification of terms such as "an upset stomach" or "a cold in the kidneys" is required. A number of reference sources are available to assist the pharmacist in deciding on the types of questions that should be asked, depending on the patient's complaint or the type of medication requested (see Appendix A). The aim of questioning is to elucidate the necessary details of the symptoms in order to screen for the appropriateness of self-treatment.

In general, the following information about the symptoms should be obtained: [8,14]

- *Location*: Where is the symptom located?
- *Quality:* What does it feel like?
- *Severity:* How severe is it?
- *Modifying Factors:* What seems to aggravate or alleviate it? Is there any particular time it occurs (e.g., on arising, after eating)?
- *Timing*: How long or how often has it been present?
- *Associated Symptoms:* Are there other, related symptoms?
- *Previous Treatment:* What has been done so far or in the past to treat this symptom? Has a physician been consulted now or in the past? If so, what happened?

In addition to gathering this information from the patient, the pharmacist should observe the patient's physical appearance (e.g., skin pallor or rash).[14]

Discussion to Prevent or Resolve Problems and Provide Information

As in prescription counseling, the pharmacist must next develop a treatment plan that may include a variety of recommendations as well as information provision.

The pharmacist must first decide if the symptoms the patient has described indicate the need for treatment. If the symptoms appear to be mild, the patient may simply need reassurance and possibly some suggestions for nondrug treatment. If the symptoms appear to be of a type, severity, and/or duration that indicate a non-self-treatable condition, the pharmacist must recommend that the patient seek the advice of a physician. Where appropriate, an interim measure may also be suggested (i.e., a nondrug treatment or temporary use of a nonprescription drug until the physician is contacted).

It is sometimes difficult for the pharmacist to make the decision to refer the patient to a physician. Five general criteria can be used to identify those patients for whom physician referral is most appropriate:[8,14]

1. *Age of the Patient.* In young children, particularly those younger than 6 months of age, conditions can change rapidly and consequences of apparently minor symptoms may be severe. Also, it is usually not possible to question the patient, and caregivers may not be observing important indicators to report. In the elderly, symptoms are often complicated by several health conditions and medications. In addition, some symptoms may be misleading, (e.g., earache is a possible symptom of angina, since pain can be referred to the neck and ear area as well as down the left arm). The elderly and very young may also react differently than the general population to certain drugs because of differences in the way they metabolize some drugs, and therefore, such patients may require adjusted dosages.

2. *Nature and Severity of Symptoms.* Symptoms such as chest pain; high fever; black, tarry stools; and colored sputum indicate severe problems that should not be self-treated. Symptoms such as pain that are reportedly quite severe should also not be self-treated.

3. *Duration of Symptoms.* Symptoms that may initially appear appropriate for self-treatment cease to be so if they continue for a prolonged time— for example, diarrhea, pain of any kind, or fever. The duration that signals a need for medical attention varies with the symptoms and with other factors, such as the age of the patient. For example, an infant should not have diarrhea for more than 24 hours, whereas an adult may tolerate it for several days without alarm.

4. *Other Existing Conditions and Medication Use.* Patients with existing chronic conditions or those taking particular types of medication may be at greater risk of complications from minor conditions than others, and therefore, should probably seek advice from their physicians for accurate assessment of their symptoms. For example, a patient with diabetes may

easily develop gangrene from a blister on his or her foot; a patient taking immunosuppressive drugs can quickly develop pneumonia from a cold. In addition, some symptoms actually may be signs of side effects or of complications of the primary condition.

Although pharmacists can certainly anticipate problems that might occur, they often do not have complete patient data to make accurate predictions, and therefore, a physician may need to be consulted. For example, for a patient with high blood pressure, an oral sympathomimetic agent would be contraindicated, but a nasal spray may be safe; unless the pharmacist had access to more detailed information about the patient's blood pressure control, he or she would be unable to make a treatment decision.

5. *Pregnancy.* There is a lack of definitive information about the teratogenic effects of drugs, and therefore, many nonprescription drugs pose a potential danger to the pregnant woman and her unborn child. In addition, there is concern that symptoms may be indicative of problems with the pregnancy, and that any treatments may stimulate contractions. Although the mother's discomfort must be balanced with concern for the developing fetus, this is best done together with the patient's physician. The pharmacist should also be alert for symptoms in a female patient that may be indicative of pregnancy, such as nausea. The pharmacist should question the patient regarding this possibility before proceeding to make a treatment recommendation.

To assist pharmacists in making these decisions, there are a number of reference guides (see Appendix A). In particular, "Handbook of Nonprescription Drugs," lists the types of questions to be considered for each class of nonprescription drugs.

If the symptoms indicate a self-treatable condition, as defined above, the treatment plan may include the recommendation of a nonprescription drug. If so, the following information should be provided regarding the nonprescription drug (as in the case of a new prescription medication):

1. *Name of the drug.*
2. *Purpose of the medication.*
3. *Directions for use.* Although they are provided on the package label, the directions for use should be pointed out to the patient, and doses should be suggested in accordance with the age of the patient. If the product requires special instructions such as insertion of eye or ear drops, this should be explained and demonstrated where appropriate.
4. *Side effects.* As in new prescription counseling, the pharmacist should preface the discussion of side effects with a mention of their rarity. The symptoms associated with possible side effects should be described, and the patient should be advised about how to avoid or deal with them (e.g., take with food to avoid stomach upset, or stop taking it if a rash develops).

5. *Precautions.* Warnings should be provided against the use of interacting medications, and where appropriate, the pharmacist should warn the patient about use of the medication during pregnancy or breast feeding, or use with alcohol.

6. *Time frame for effectiveness.* The patient should be advised of the time frame within which the treatment should take effect—for example, a few days for a bulk laxative or immediately for a glycerin suppository. A patient equipped with this information will be less likely to discontinue treatment before it has had time to take effect or, conversely, to persist with a treatment that is ineffective.

Regardless of whether or not a product is being recommended, the treatment plan should include provision of information about the condition and symptoms.

1. *Advice regarding symptoms.* Since self-treated symptoms should be self-limiting and mild, recommendations for nonprescription drug use, nondrug treatment, or no treatment at all should always be accompanied by a suggested time limit for specified outcomes beyond which they should consult a physician. As with prescription counseling, these outcomes should be discussed with the patient and measurable indicators should be agreed on to determine if the treatment is appropriate and effective. The time limit will vary for each type of symptom. For example, for diarrhea, medical advice should be sought after a few days, but for cold symptoms, advice should be sought only after a few weeks.

   In addition, the patient should be told that certain changes in the original symptoms could indicate a more serious underlying condition that should be reported to the physician (e.g., changes such as the appearance of blood in diarrhea).

   Patients should also be warned that continual or repeated use of a nonprescription medication may alleviate symptoms, but may mask more serious conditions. If symptoms such as abdominal pain, headaches, or indigestion recur frequently, they may be indicative of serious conditions.

2. *Advice regarding the condition.* Information may also be provided about the condition itself and about measures the patient can take to prevent further contagion or recurrence.

3. *Nondrug treatment.* Where appropriate, the pharmacist should include in the treatment plan advice regarding other self-care treatments, such as use of a humidifier and increased fluid intake to reduce congestion.

References are available to assist the pharmacist in providing such information to the patient (see Appendix A).

Closing Discussion
As in prescription drug counseling, the nonprescription-drug-counseling encounter should end with a summary of important points and an attempt to get

feedback from the patient to make sure that there are no misunderstandings. The patient should be encouraged to ask questions, whether at that time or later. If print information about the condition or medication is available, it may be given to the patient.

If the pharmacist has a patient record for that patient, he or she may make a record of the nonprescription drug purchase. Informing the patient that a record will be made may increase the patient's trust in both the pharmacist's counseling and the pharmacy's record-keeping services.

A self-care documenting form has been proposed to allow the pharmacist to record the encounter for his or her own records, a copy of which can be given to the patient for a written reminder of the pharmacist's recommendations. Although it may take time to complete the form, it provides continuity of care for subsequent encounters with the patient, improved management of potential liability, and promotion of a perception in the patient's mind that a valuable health service is being provided.[5] Because the patient's medication history is part of any decisions made by the pharmacist, the medication history (a printout from the patient's computer record or a form filled out at the time) should be attached to the documentation. An example of a Nonprescription Counseling Form is provided in Appendix C.

Follow-up Discussion
The pharmacist should also encourage a follow-up consultation to ensure that the patient's symptoms are diminishing and that the medication is effective and is being used appropriately. At that time, the pharmacist can ensure that appropriate outcomes are occurring and can make further recommendations.

The Medication-History Interview
Conducting a medication-history interview with a new patient is an important activity in both the hospital and the community-pharmacy settings. Community pharmacists often complain that it is difficult to counsel patients, because they don't know the patients' medical history or details of the conditions being treated.

Pharmacists in a hospital or clinic setting usually have the benefit of the patient's medical chart for reference. The chart will provide information regarding the condition or symptoms for which the medication has been prescribed, other existing conditions, and any medications the patient is currently using or has used in the past. With future developments such as 'smart cards' and interactive computer links, community pharmacists will gain access to more patient data. In some locations today, it is possible to gain access through a computer to lists of medications dispensed at any pharmacy for a particular patient.

This information, however, does not provide complete information regarding actual medication use. The information in the patient chart was most likely gathered by a physician or a nurse, both of whom would not have been concerned with medication use. In addition, such records are often completed by several providers, who differ in the amount and type of information they record and in the terms they use, and therefore, may be incomplete and confusing.[18]

In order to gather complete information regarding medication use, the pharmacist needs to interact with the patient and gain some understanding of his or her existing or potential concerns about, and problems with, medication use. The pharmacist is best able to gather this information, as studies have demonstrated that pharmacists generally gain more detailed information than physicians or nurses during a medication-history interview.[19, 20] Therefore, whether or not medical records are available for reference, it is important for the pharmacist to conduct a medication-history interview with the patient.

However, if the patient's medical record is not available, the pharmacist may need to supplement patient-provided information by contacting the physician. Patients have been found to be fairly knowledgeable and accurate in reporting health and functional status and medication use. There are, however, some areas that they often do not fully understand or about which they may not have been informed, for example, the types of laboratory test or even some major hospital procedures they have undergone or their results.[18]

Although pharmacists usually gather a certain amount of information from patients (such as personal information, chronic conditions, and allergies), they often do not conduct complete medication-history interviews because of time constraints. Conducting a complete interview of this sort is admittedly a time-consuming process. To save time, the patient can be asked to complete a written medication-history questionnaire. The pharmacist can discuss the information privately with the patient afterwards, probing to gather complete details and inquiring about any concerns or problems the patient may have. A sample of this sort of questionnaire is reproduced in Appendix C.

OBRA-'90 requires that certain patient information be gathered for Medicaid patients, but it is recommended that this service be provided to all patients.[1]

Goals of the Medication-History Interview

The main purpose of the medication-history interview is to assist the pharmacist in identifying real and potential problems with current and newly prescribed medications. It also provides a basis for the ongoing assessment of the patient's medication use. Specific information about the conditions being treated and the medications used in the past and present will help the pharmacist to evaluate the appropriateness of the types and dosages of current and newly prescribed drugs. In addition, it will assist the pharmacist in evaluating the effectiveness of past and current treatments.

Information gathered in the medication history will also help the pharmacist to detect other real and potential problems associated with current or new medications such as drug–drug interactions, drug–disease interactions, side effects, adverse effects, allergies, or noncompliance. Further questioning of the patient can expose the factors contributing to these problems, such as misunderstandings or double doctoring, and possible solutions to these problems.

This information and information about the patient's occupation, language level, and perhaps attitudes and biases may also contribute to understanding and solving drug-related problems. Such information also allows the pharmacist to assess the patient's needs for future counseling and education.

The interaction with the patient that the medication-history interview affords will help to create a helping relationship between the pharmacist and patient, which is an important part in the pharmaceutical care process.[2]

The information gathered in the medication-history interview will also assist the pharmacist in conducting an informed discussion with the patient's physician if the need arises.

Finally, conducting a medication-history interview allows the pharmacist to promote a "value-added" service offered by the pharmacy. Patients should be made aware that this interview is of benefit to them and to their optimal health care, and that it is an added service provided by this particular pharmacy. This may encourage the patient to become a loyal customer, feeling that he is now "registered" at this pharmacy that offers "extra" services.

A summary of the goals of the medication-history interview is found in Table 5.1.

Table 5.1   Goals of the Medication-History Interview

1. *To provide a basis for ongoing assessment of medication use*

2. *To evaluate the appropriateness of the drugs selected and the dosing prescribed*

3. *To evaluate the effectiveness of past, current, and newly prescribed medications*

4. *To assist the pharmacist in identifying other potential and actual problems associated with current or newly prescribed medications such as drug–drug interactions, drug–disease interactions, side effects, adverse effects, allergies, and noncompliance*

5. *To identify factors contributing to these problems and their possible solutions*

6. *To allow the pharmacist to assess the patient's needs for future counseling and education*

7. *To assist the pharmacist in conducting informed discussions with the physician*

8. *To help create a helping relationship between the pharmacist and patient*

9. *To provide an "extra" service offered by the pharmacy to gain customer loyalty*

Conducting the Interview

Figure 5.2 illustrates the suggested flow for a complete medication-history interview. Careful probing is necessary to gather complete data, while preventing an atmosphere of inquisition from developing and allowing plenty of time for the patient to respond to questions.[19] Communication skills involved with questioning and probing will be discussed in Chapter 7, and a suggested dialogue is presented in Appendix B.

The suggested protocol is recommended because it structures questioning in a logical sequence that helps the patient recall events and assists the pharmacist in assessing the information gathered. By staying on track, the pharmacist will be less likely to miss necessary information. The patient, however, may want to make comments or ask questions, and this input should not be ignored by the pharmacist. The patient's concerns may either be discussed briefly at the time (if they pertain to the information being gathered) or politely deferred until the end of the interview.

The pharmacist should resist making recommendations or giving advice until after the interview has ended and a complete assessment has been made of the data gathered.

Since personal data will be discussed during the interview, it is necessary to conduct it in a private setting—a separate cubicle or office.[19] If neither is available, the interview may have to be conducted over the telephone at a later time.

The Interview Protocol

Opening Discussion

The opening should set the tone for the interview. It is particularly important to develop a helping relationship with the patient in order to make him or her feel comfortable and better prepared for a discussion of personal information.

The opening consists of a greeting and introduction by the pharmacist, and a check on the identity of the patient. If appropriate —for example, in a clinic or a hospital setting—the pharmacist might explain that he or she is working together with the physician. A few minutes should be allowed for casual conversation to set the patient at ease and to further develop a helping relationship. Topics such as the weather or the patient's family might be briefly discussed.

The purpose of the interview and the type of information to be gathered should be explained—in terms of the benefits to the patient and *not* for the convenience of the pharmacist. The pharmacist should explain that information about the patient's conditions and medication use will be gathered to get a complete picture of his or her situation and to help the pharmacist ensure that the patient is getting the most effective therapy possible. The pharmacist might also explain that he or she will be checking for any problems the patient may have had in the past with drug use (such as drug interactions). At this point, it is important to assure the patient that all information gathered is strictly confidential.

Figure 5.2
Flow Chart For Medication-History Interview

Opening Discussion
• Introduction   • Explain purpose   • Insure confidentiality
↓

Inquiry of Personal Information
• Age, Occupation, etc.   • Use of health care professionals and attitudes
↓

Discussion of Medical Conditions and Medications Use

Condition No. 1
• Name or symptom of condition   • How long?
↓

Current Medications for Condition No. 1
Medication A
• Name of medication
• Who prescribed it?
• How is it taken? (specifics)
• Does it help?
• If noncompliance detected,
• What are its causes?
• Side effects and adverse effects

Repeat Questions About Each Medication
↓

Past Medications for Condition No. 1
• Names of medication   • Reasons for discontinuing use

Repeat Questions About Current and Past Medications for Each Condition
↓

Nonprescription Drug Use
• Name
• Usage—why, when, how used, how long?
• Side effects and adverse effect
• Effectiveness

Discussion of Alcohol and Tobacco Use
↓

Discussion of Drug Sensitivity
↓

Closing Discussion
↓

Follow-up Discussions

The pharmacist should try to impress on the patient the importance of complete and correct information in the interests of an accurate pharmaceutical assessment. The approximate length of the interview should also be mentioned. The pharmacist should then allow the patient to give consent to continue. This sets the stage for co-operation between the pharmacist and the patient because they have mutually agreed to proceed with the interview.

Personal Information

A certain amount of personal information needs to be gathered including name, address, and health-insurance information. The patient's age (birth date) and occupation should also be obtained, because this information might affect the selection of treatments in the future. The names of the patient's physicians and other health-care personnel, such as a chiropractor or ophthalmologist, should also be noted. This will help to suggest the direction of further questions about all pertinent conditions, treatments, and medications (traditional and nontraditional). The information will be useful if the need arises to contact these other health professionals to gather more complete information or to discuss identified problems.

During this questioning, the patient should be asked a general question about any difficulties accessing necessary care, (e.g., difficulty reaching the physician, difficulty paying for care, difficulty getting help at home for health care). This may indicate a source of medication use behaviors or problems.

Discussion of Medical Conditions and Medication Use

To help the patient recall details about conditions and medications, it is suggested that each condition and the drugs associated with it be dealt with separately before proceeding to the next condition.

The name of each condition or a description of the symptoms associated with it should be ascertained at the outset. As discussed, the patient's knowledge in this area may not be complete, and the pharmacist may have to supplement data gathered from the patient with information obtained from other sources, such as the medical record or the physician, if possible.

The patient should also be questioned about the duration of the condition, since this may elicit the patient's concerns or any misunderstandings about the condition.

The patient should then be asked what medications he or she is using for the particular condition, and the following information should be gathered about each medication separately:

1. *Name of the medication.* If the patient does not know the name of the drug, the pharmacist can ask the patient to describe it or show it. Alternatively, the pharmacist can arrange to telephone the patient later.
2. *Name of the prescriber.* Obtaining the name of the prescribing physician will help reduce the possibility of duplicate prescriptions by specialists and family doctors.

3. *How the medication is used.* The patient should be questioned about specific details pertaining to dosage, frequency of use on a day-to-day basis, and the times during the day when the medication is taken. Information should also be gathered about food consumption in relation to medication use. If noncompliance is evident from the patient's responses to these questions, the pharmacist should probe to determine how frequently doses are missed or improperly taken.
4. *Duration of use.*
5. *Efficacy of the medication.* The patient should be asked whether, in his or her opinion, the medication is helping to alleviate the symptoms. If the patient perceives the prescribed drug to be ineffective, the pharmacist should ask the patient how the drug is ineffective and whether there are any times or circumstances that seem to make the drug more or less effective.
6. *Compliance investigation.* If information about the use of medication points to noncompliance, it is important to determine its possible causes. As discussed in Chapter 4, the reasons may be varied, and careful but thorough probing may be required to uncover them. The patient may be asked directly (but, again, in a nonconfrontational manner) about his failure to take the medication in the dose and frequency recommended. Suggested dialogue is provided in Appendix B.
7. *Side effects and adverse effects.* The patient should be asked about any problems experienced with medication use. A general question about such problems may be followed by probing for specific symptoms (reported in the literature), the details of which—severity, frequency, duration, and other related factors—should be gathered.

After all medications used for a particular condition have been ascertained, the patient should be asked about past medications used for this condition. If possible, the pharmacist should try to determine the names of the medications and the reasons why they were discontinued. The patient may not recall this information, and other sources of data may need to be used. This information will help the pharmacist make recommendations to the physician about alternative therapies, if necessary.

The pharmacist should proceed in sequence with each condition and its associated medications. The pharmacist should then ask generally whether any other prescription medications are being used. This provides a check for things forgotten and for any medications the patient may be taking that aren't necessarily related to a particular condition (such as prescribed vitamins).

Discussion of Nonprescription Medication Use

It is important to gather information about self-treatment by the patient, because nonprescription medications may interact with prescribed drugs or interfere with diagnostic tests. In addition, the patient may be using them to treat previously undisclosed side effects of prescribed medications.

The patient should be asked a general question about the use of the medications that he or she purchases, followed by probing to prompt his or her memory. For example, the pharmacist might mention the categories of nonprescription drugs or their uses—medicine to treat coughs and colds, upset stomach, etc.

The same details should be gathered about nonprescription medications as prescribed medications, including the name of the drug, the reason for use, the dosage and frequency of use, duration of use, effectiveness, and any possible side effects.

Discussion of Alcohol and Tobacco Use

Since alcohol and tobacco use can affect certain medications and conditions, it is important to include information pertaining to them in a medication history. This topic is more personal than that of medication use, and therefore should be introduced with tact, in a nonjudgmental manner. Suggested wording is provided in Appendix B. The pharmacist should explain that this information is important since alcohol or tobacco may affect therapy. If the patient is taking medications that have the potential to interact with alcohol, the pharmacist should also inquire whether medication use is altered when the patient consumes alcoholic beverages.

Discussion of Drug Sensitivity

The pharmacist should inquire whether the patient knows of any medications to which he or she may be allergic. Since the patient may not be aware of specific allergies, he or she should also be asked more generally if he or she has ever experienced an unpleasant reaction to a medication.

If the patient reports an allergy or adverse reactions, the pharmacist should ask for a description of the effects experienced. This will allow him or her to evaluate whether the reaction was a genuine sensitivity to the medication or simply a side effect. For example, although people often report that they are allergic to ASA, further questioning reveals that what they experience is stomach discomfort—a side effect of acetylsalicylic acid rather than an allergic reaction to it. In addition, the pharmacist should ask whether the patient has informed his or her prescribing physician of the problem, and if not, recommend he or she do so.

Closing Discussion

In closing the medication history interview, the pharmacist should offer the patient an opportunity to add any information that might not already have been covered. The pharmacist might simply ask "Is there anything else that you'd like to tell me about?"

The pharmacist should explain to the patient that the information will be included with his or her patient record for future reference, and that it may be discussed with the physician if any problems develop in the course of the therapy. Confidentiality may be stressed once more.

If a medication is being dispensed at this time, the pharmacist will assess the data immediately and proceed with the drug counseling. If a medication is not being dispensed at this time, the patient may be told that the pharmacist will review the data to assess the drug therapy and that the pharmacist will discuss it further at an arranged time.

At this time, the pharmacist may wish to give the patient his or her business card and offer to answer questions or discuss concerns any time. This will help to develop a relationship with the patient, as well as promote the services of the pharmacy.

Finally, the patient should be thanked for visiting the pharmacy.

Assessment and Documentation

Having gathered a considerable amount of information from the patient, the pharmacist must next assess the data in order to achieve the goals of the exercise as discussed above. Each medication should be evaluated to detect any existing or potential problems with existing or new medication. In particular, the pharmacist should evaluate medication appropriateness and effectiveness. The data should also be reviewed for evidence of medication problems such as noncompliance, drug–drug interactions, drug–disease interactions, side effects, adverse effects, or history of drug sensitivity.

If necessary, the pharmacist should consult reference texts to evaluate these problems and to determine the appropriate course of action. On reflection, it may be apparent that certain additional data are necessary, such as results of laboratory tests, in which case these data should be retrieved.

The results of this assessment should then be documented by the pharmacist noting specific problems, possible causes, recommended action, and treatment plan. The pharmacist should also assess the patient's need for future counseling and education. If noncompliance has been detected, the information gathered concerning reasons associated with it must be considered and along with possible ways to treat the problem, as discussed in Chapter 4. If the patient has raised certain concerns or questions or has demonstrated a lack of understanding about his or her condition or medication, plans to provide information should be made.

Follow-Up

The pharmacist should next consider the course of action that must be taken as a follow-up to the medical-history interview. It may include the following measures:

1. Contacting the physician to inform him or her of any problems with the medication detected and to discuss the treatment of these problems.
2. Recommending to the physician that the prescribed therapy be discontinued or altered and suggesting possible alternatives.
3. Recommending to the patient ways of using the medication that will improve compliance and, consequently, the effectiveness of the therapy (e.g., suggesting the use of memory aids).

4. Applying various techniques to overcome noncompliance (e.g., reminding the patient of the importance of the medication to the outcome of the condition).
5. Recommending to the patient methods for reducing side effects (e.g., taking the medication with food).

Any such actions taken should be documented and the outcomes of those actions documented (e.g., discussion with the physician concerning the patient's experience of side effects resulted in a reduction of the dose to a specific level).

Follow-up should also be made with the patient to assess the effectiveness of any recommendations.

Using the preceding guidelines, the pharmacist in the situation discussed at the beginning of this chapter would have been more successful in her task as illustrated.

Alternate Situation

Pharmacist: Hello, Mrs. Hampton. Is this your first time here at our pharmacy?

Patient: Yes, I usually go to the pharmacy close to my office.

Pharmacist: Well, we're happy to help you here today. Do you live nearby?

Patient: Yes, just down River Street.

Pharmacist: Oh, yes, I know that street. It's a nice area. Well, I hope we'll see more of you. Before I get your prescription ready, I want to explain to you that in this pharmacy we keep records about you and the medications you take to help ensure that you get the most benefit from them. To start your record, I'd like to ask you for some information about your health conditions and any current medication use. Of course, this information is strictly confidential. To save time, perhaps you could fill out this patient history form while we prepare your prescription. Then, I'll discuss it with you when your prescription is ready, in about 10 minutes.

Patient: Yes, all right, but doesn't my doctor have this information?

Pharmacist: Your doctor may have some of this information, but we don't have access to that information. We need to check for any problems with certain medications, for example allergies or interactions between medications.

Patient: Oh, I see. I'll have to think for a minute to remember all this.

Pharmacist: Take your time. It's important that the information is as accurate as can be.

...10 minutes pass

Pharmacist: Mrs. Hampton. Your prescription is ready now. Will you come in here where we can speak more privately *(indicates counseling booth).*

Patient: *(comes into booth and hands over the patient history form)* Here's the form.

Pharmacist: Thanks for completing that for me. As I said, this will help us to provide the best care for you. I'll just take a few minutes to review it.

Patient: OK.

Pharmacist: Now, let me see. *(reads over the patient history form)* You've filled in just about everything. You didn't list any nonprescription medications. Sometimes people don't think of things like vitamins as nonprescription medications. Do you take any vitamins?

Patient: Oh, yes, you're right. I didn't think of that as medication. I take those calcium tablets over there *(indicates a particular brand and strength)*.

Pharmacist: I see. And can you tell me how you take them?

Patient: Three tablets every morning like clock-work.

Pharmacist: Good for you. Now, how about anything else, like ... *(proceeds to explore each category of nonprescription drug and discovers that the patient uses a popular antacid. The pharmacist proceeds to ask about dosage and frequency. Following that, the pharmacist asks a few more questions to fill in gaps in data, then closes the discussion)* Well, I think I have the complete information now. Is there anything else that you'd like to mention?

Patient: No, I don't think so.

Pharmacist: OK then, thank you for helping me. I'll be keeping that information in our records so we can refer to it when you come in for any other medications. In fact, it has been helpful already in uncovering some possible problems with getting the most benefit from your new medication. Let's talk about that now.

Patient: *(sounding interested)* Yes, all right.

Pharmacist: What did the doctor tell you about your prescription?

Patient: She told me to take one capsule every 6 hours.

Pharmacist: That's right. And did she explain how it will help you?

Patient: Not really. It's for my skin. I seem to be going through a second puberty, because pimples are breaking out on my face and back.

Pharmacist: This is an antibiotic to treat infections. In this case, it seems to cut down on the number and severity of pustules developing. You need to take it regularly to keep the pimples under control.

Patient: Oh, I see.

Pharmacist: *(proceeds to explain how to take it in relation to meals, etc.)* Now, I mentioned that there was a potential problem. The calcium tablets and the antacid you take can interfere with how well the tetracycline is absorbed into your body from your stomach and decrease how well it works. You shouldn't take them within 1 hour of the tetracycline.

Patient: Oh, really?

Pharmacist: *(proceeds to discuss scheduling these medications to avoid problems)* Do you see any difficulty in taking it like this?

Patient: No, I think I can keep track of that. I have a pretty good memory.

Pharmacist: Good. Now, did the doctor tell you anything to watch out for while you're on this?

Patient: No, not that I can remember.

Pharmacist: Sometimes people find these medications make them more sensitive to the sunlight. Do you take part in any outdoor activities?

Patient: I go for walks some evenings and on the weekend.

Pharmacist: Just avoid getting too much sun or wear a sunscreen to be safe. There's a few other things you should read about here on this information sheet *(points to appropriate section on information sheet)*. People very rarely experience these side effects and they probably won't happen to you, but if you should notice anything unusual, let your doctor or a pharmacist know right away. There are a few other things here about how to store the medication, etc. You can read this information when you get home.

Patient: OK.

Pharmacist: The doctor hasn't indicated any further refills. Did she explain what to do when you finish the medication?

Patient: Yes, I have an appointment to see her in about 1 month, when these pills are gone.

Pharmacist: You should be seeing an effect by then. Do you have any questions about all this?

Patient: No, I think it's clear.

Pharmacist: Good. I'll call you in 1 week to see how things are going.

Patient: That would be nice.

Pharmacist: Thank you for your time today. Call me if you have any questions or concerns. Here's my card.

Patient: OK. Thank you. *(walks away thinking)* This is great! I'll come to this pharmacy from now on since they have my record. *(when she gets home she reads over the information sheet and posts the pharmacist's business card on the bulletin board by the phone for future reference)*

Further Discussion

In this situation, the pharmacist was able to complete the medication history and the counseling as well as establish a relationship with the patient for the future. By introducing the need for the medication history, as well as introducing the medication counseling, the pharmacist gained the cooperation of the patient and was able to complete her task successfully.

Summary

The protocols for patient counseling suggested in this chapter are of course simply a guideline to help pharmacists organize their thoughts, and to be as efficient and effective as possible. Often it is difficult or perhaps inappropriate to follow these protocols. The need for adjustments and the ways that counseling content may be adjusted will be the subject of Chapter 8.

Since these protocols suggest that the patient and the pharmacist should be involved in the counseling discussion, pharmacists require skills in communication to engage the patient as well as to be sure that both the patient and pharmacist understand each other.[19] Communication skills for patient counseling will be reviewed in Chapter 7. Suggested pharmacist dialogues to assist the pharmacist in phrasing introductions and questions during counseling are provided in Appendix B.

The counseling protocols suggested often involve presenting the patient with large amounts of information. Using various educational techniques and counseling aids can assist pharmacists to be efficient and effective in counseling. This will be the topic of the following chapter.

References

1. Feegel K, Dix Smith M. Counseling and cognitive services for Medicaid patients under OBRA-'90. Pharm Times. 1992;9 Supp:1-9.
2. Strand LM, Cipolle RJ, Morley PC. Pharmaceutical care: an introduction. Current Concepts, 1992. Kalamazoo, MI The Upjohn Co. 1992:15.
3. Anon. The pharmacy patient's Bill of Rights. US Pharm. 1992:(5):61-68
4. Levin LS. Self-medication: The social perspective. Self-Medication: The New Era...A Symposium. Washington, DC: The Proprietary Association. 1980.
5. Srnka QM. Implementing a self-care-consulting practice. Am Pharm. 1993;NS33(1):61-69.
6. Holt GA, Hall EL. The self-care movement. In: Handbook of Non-Prescription Drugs. 9th ed. Washington, DC: American Pharmaceutical Association. 1990.
7. Johnson R, Pope C. Health status and social factors in non-prescribed drug use. Med Care. 1983;21:225-233.
8. Boyce R, Herrier R. Obtaining and using patient data. Am Pharm. 1991;NS31(7):65-70
9. Segal M. Rx OTC...The switch is on. FDA Consumer, March, 1991.
10. Rantucci M, Segal HJ. Hazardous non-prescription analgesic use by the elderly. J Soc Admin Pharm. 1991;8(3):108-120.
11. Colt H, Shapiro A. Drug-induced illness as a cause for admission to a community hospital. J Am Ger Soc.1989;37(4):323-326.
12. Salerno E, Ries D, Sank J, et al. Self-medication behaviors. Fla J Hosp Pharm. 1985;5(7):13-28.
13. Wilkinson I, Darby D, Mant A. Self-care and self-medication: An evaluation of individual's health care decisions. Med Care 1987;25(10):965-978.
14. Klein-Schwartz W, Hoopes JM. Patient assessment and consultation. In: Handbook of Non-Prescription Drugs. 9th ed. Washington, DC.: American Pharmaceutical Association, 1990.
15. Penna R. Introduction. In: Handbook of Non-Prescription Drugs. 5th ed. Washington, DC.: American Pharmaceutical Association,1977.
16. Schering Laboratories. The pharmacist as an OTC consultant. The Schering Report (1980). Kenilworth, NJ: Schering Laboratories. 1980.
17. Anon. Availability of RPh Governs patron's drug store choice. Am Druggist.1985;192(3):52-54.

18. Betz Brown J, Adams M. Patients as reliable reporters of medical care process. Med Care. 1992;30(5):400-411.
19. Covington T, Whitney Jr H. Patient-pharmacist communication techniques. Drug Intell Clin Pharm. 1971;5(11):370-76.
20. Gurwich E. Comparison of medication histories acquired by pharmacists and physicians. Am J Hosp Pharm. 1983;40:1541-1542.

6
EDUCATIONAL METHODS AND COUNSELING AIDS

Patients have varied wants and needs regarding education and counseling. Consider the following patients' comments:

Patient A: I like talking to my pharmacist. She usually does more than just give me information about my medication.

Patient B: I don't have time to stay in the pharmacy talking to the pharmacist. Can't I get information about my medication some other way?

Patient C: I like to have lots of detailed information about my condition and my medication. Is there some way I can review this information at home?

Patient D: I don't read English very well. Is there some way I can get information to take home?

Patient E: I take so many different medications that sometimes it's hard to keep them all straight. The pharmacist tells me how to take them, but when I get home I get confused. Sometimes I forget whether I've taken something or not.

Pharmacists often find it difficult to meet the needs of all these patients. When pharmacists think of counseling patients and providing information, they generally think only of talking to the patient (often in a lecture format rather than a discussion) or providing written information. However, a number of methods are available to provide counseling and education. Knowledge of these methods and aids can assist pharmacists in conducting effective and efficient patient counseling. In addition, as discussed in Chapter 4, compliance can be improved by the use of counseling aids. Pharmacists need to be able to develop a plan for each patient using a selection of the available counseling methods and aids.

Educational Methods

Studies of education have found that many possible methods exist for facilitating learning other than the traditional lecture-style presentation. As patient counseling has gained acceptance as a role for pharmacists, more and better materials and resources have become available. Pharmacists can employ a range of educational methods with their patients, from lectures, dialogue and discussion, and print information, to audiovisual methods, demonstrations (and practice) of techniques, video simulations, and computer-assisted learning.

Lectures

Lectures represent the traditional style of presenting information.[1] Although pharmacists often employ this approach on a one-to-one basis, lectures should really be limited to larger groups, for example community groups, where individual discussion is not possible.

Although not all pharmacists are comfortable with the idea of lecturing to the public, pharmacists should attempt to promote themselves to their communities as public speakers on health and medication topics. Speaking to community groups is one of the best ways to gain public trust for the profession and to serve clients.[2] Involvement in lecturing will not only promote the profession of pharmacy, and the individual pharmacist in the community, but may also provide the pharmacist with greater confidence in speaking to patients on an individual basis. Pharmacists in institutional settings are often called on to address groups of patients or health professionals, and therefore should become comfortable with this method.

Various books and courses are available to assist pharmacists in developing their public-speaking skills and lecturing techniques. [2-5] Tips for planning, organizing, preparing for, and presenting a speech should be reviewed by pharmacists planning such presentations. This will be discussed in more detail later in this chapter.

Because lecture material is often considered boring and because retention is generally fairly low, lectures should incorporate other educational techniques such as audiovisual aids and group discussion (e.g., a question-and-answer period at the end of the presentation). Descriptions of personal experiences and discussion of particular cases help audiences identify with the material being presented and may increase the impact on behavior and attitude.[3]

Since the learner/patient is passive in the lecture situation, there is little opportunity for the pharmacist to address individual concerns or to have much effect on one patient's understanding or attitudes. Because the pharmacist wants to improve the patient's behavior and attitudes as well as his or her knowledge, a lecture is not recommended for counseling one patient.

Dialogue and Discussion

Although lecturing is a useful skill to develop, one-on-one dialogue with the patient through a patient-counseling protocol as described in the previous chapter is the essence of the pharmacist's regular duties.

The discussion may be guided by the pharmacist, but should allow for as much participation as possible by the patient. Herrier said that "when pharmacists consult with patients it's like they push a button, turn on the tape recorder, and recite the prescription directions like a machine."[6] He recommends that pharmacists use techniques that allow the patient to be involved in the patient-counseling discussion so that the pharmacist can find out what the patient knows and/or needs to know.[6] Communication techniques to encourage discussion during patient counseling will be discussed in Chapter 7, and suggested dialogues for patient counseling that promote discussion are shown in Appendix B.

Although the dialogue-and-discussion approach may be more time-consuming than simply presenting a lecture, it is more effective in improving the patient's understanding of medication use and in altering his or her attitudes. In one study of various counseling methods, one group of patients received information via the standard instructions and accessory labels simply read by the pharmacist, whereas another group of patients received the same instructions plus a personal consultation with the pharmacist.[7] Patients receiving the consultation not only had a greater understanding of their medication (identifying appropriate administration times, special instructions, side effects, what to do if they missed a dose), but also were more compliant.[7]

Discussion does not necessarily have to be conducted face-to-face and can be conducted over the telephone. In the above study, patients who received no oral consultation at the time of dispensing received telephone consultation as a follow-up on the fourth or fifth day of therapy. This improved compliance to the same degree that the face-to-face consultation had in the other group.[7]

A discussion may include more than one learner—perhaps the patient's family members or several patients with similar problems. Involvement of friends or family members in the patient-education discussion may help them to support the patient and as a result, enhance the patient's medication attitudes and behaviors as discussed in Chapters 3 and 4. Discussion among patients with similar concerns can also improve their medication attitudes and behaviors.

Print Information

Print information is often used by pharmacists as a substitute for patient counseling. OBRA-'90 specifies that written information may not take the place of counseling, although it may be used to supplement the pharmacist's verbal instructions.[8] When used alone, print information about specific drugs or conditions is of limited effectiveness in improving patients' knowledge.[9] Print information alone may in fact create certain misunderstandings through ambiguous language that requires further explanation (e.g., avoid prolonged exposure to sunlight; take with meals).

Print information in conjunction with dialogue and discussion, however, has been found to be more effective than verbal methods alone.[10] Discussion allows the pharmacist to clarify written language and to receive feedback from the patient regarding his or her level of understanding. The print information can then be taken home and read at the patient's leisure. In the pharmacy, the patient often feels rushed or overwhelmed with information or emotions. Elderly people, in particular, often feel the need for more time to absorb the information provided by the pharmacist.[11] After reading the print information, the patient is generally able to identify areas that need clarification, which can then be achieved through further dialogue with the pharmacist.

Studies find that the majority of patients prefer written and verbal information in combination, although it is an individual decision.[12,13] In one study, although 45% of patients preferred both a leaflet and pharmacist counseling, 30% preferred counseling alone, and 20% preferred the leaflet alone; younger patients (31 to 55 years of age) were more likely to prefer the leaflet.[12] In another study, although 65% of patients preferred a combination of written and verbal information, patients with higher education level or receiving refill medication were more likely to prefer written information only.[13] These patients may have believed that they did not need the additional verbal information (although this may not reflect their actual needs), or that the verbal information may have been poorly presented.

Print information may be provided to the patient in a variety of forms, including the required prescription label, auxiliary labels, information sheets, pamphlets, or booklets. Appendix A lists available information resources designed specifically for provision to patients. Some of these resources may be available in a variety of languages, as well as in larger print for patients with impaired vision.

As well as preprinted information resources, many computer programs are available that can print medication information at the time of dispensing and personalize it for the patient (see Appendix A).[14,15]

Any print information given to the patient should be scrutinized by the pharmacist to ensure that it contains appropriate information that reflects and reinforces the information provided verbally. The pharmacist should check that the language is clear, and free of vague instructions such as "plenty of water." The language should be at an appropriate level, free of jargon or technical terminology, and the layout and print size should be easy to read.

The reading level of print material is of particular concern. An estimated 13% to 40% of Americans are illiterate, and 20% are marginally literate; so comprehension cannot be taken for granted.[14] These people generally are English speaking, have had some formal education, are likely to be long-time unemployed, and are younger than 40 years of age, (although 26% of native-born Americans over 60 apparently cannot read).[15] People who do read generally read at one or two grade levels below their last completed grade at school. Thus, the general public reads at about the grade 7 or 8 level. In spite of this, materials on medication and other health topics are often found to require greater than grade 8 level, some even requiring at least a college education. In one review of 111 patient-oriented brochures and pamphlets, 50% were written above the grade 8 level.[16,17]

This underscores the importance of using print information only in conjunction with dialogue and discussion to clarify meanings. In addition, pharmacists preparing their own print materials should consider readability. Some guidelines for preparing and evaluating patient-education materials will be provided later in this chapter.

Audiovisual Aids

Many people find learning easier when they can see or hear information.[1] Information presented in the form of diagrams or pictures can, therefore, improve the patient's understanding of the method of application or ingestion of medications. Audiotapes or videotapes may also improve understanding and help alter attitudes about medication use and illness. For example, a video simulation of a patient using an inhaler may be helpful in changing other patients' attitudes about the need for correct use, and in improving their confidence about using the medication properly. Seeing patients similar to themselves develop skills or wrestle with concerns and problems with medication similar to their own may be more persuasive than having a health professional present information.

Patients may find audiotapes more interesting or easier to comprehend than reading material, particularly if they are vision impaired. In addition, the professional presenter in an audiotape or videotape may be a more persuasive speaker than the pharmacist.

Audiovisual aids may be used with one patient or with small groups of patients. Like print information, these aids tend to be most effective when combined with discussion with the patient before or after the presentation.[18]

A growing selection of audiovisual materials are available, including sound and slide shows, videotapes, audiotapes, and even comic books. Tapes on specific drugs, diseases, and devices (e.g., inhalers, injection devices) are available. A list of some audiovisual materials currently available can be found in Appendix A.

Although these materials may be expensive to produce initially, they are used repeatedly, and may be cost-effective in terms of saving pharmacist or physician time.[18] Reports of the use of audiovisual programs for patient counseling suggest that they are well received by patients and can indeed be effective in improving patient knowledge and skills as well as patient satisfaction.[19-24] Some studies show audiovisual materials to be equivalent to verbal counseling in improving patient knowledge, however, like print information, these aids tend to be most effective when combined with discussion with the patient before or after the presentation.[18,19]

A viewing area can be set up in the pharmacy, in the waiting area, or preferably in an area with some privacy. Patients may also be allowed to take audiovisual material home and on return to discuss it with the pharmacist to clarify and discuss any new issues.

As with print information, audiovisual materials should be reviewed and evaluated by the pharmacist to determine if the material is appropriate for the particular patient. Criteria for evaluating patient education videotapes will be presented later in this chapter.

Demonstrations and Practice of Techniques

When a medication requires a particular technique of administration, such as inhalation or injection, demonstration by the pharmacist or by videotape is an effective method of patient education. This approach clarifies procedures, since it is easier to follow than verbal instruction alone. When patients are also given the opportunity to practice the technique, they can develop the requisite skill. By observing the patient practicing, the pharmacist can detect possible errors and subsequently correct them.

Studies show demonstration and practice to be superior to written instruction in this type of situation. In a study of patients given metered-dose inhalers for the first time, patients were personally instructed by a pharmacist using a placebo inhaler and instruction sheet or by videotape then allowed a further 5 minutes to become familiar with inhaler use. These patients performed significantly better than those provided only with written instructions when asked to demonstrate inhaler use 10 minutes and 2 weeks later.[19]

Computer-Assisted Patient Education

With the increased availability and ease of development of software, computers have become another educational method to aid pharmacists in providing patients with general health information as well as information about specific health and medication topics. As early as 1986, computer software was available for use by patients in the United States.[25] Topics may include good health habits, poison information, specific disease information, drug information on common medications, and deciding when to seek medical care.[25] Computer-assisted programs are also available to assist pharmacists in providing information.

In a trial of a computer-assisted lesson on general drug knowledge, a quiz format allowed patients to test their knowledge then read information that they did not know.[26] Users evaluated the computer program favorably (86% responding that they learned something useful), and an evaluation of test responses showed improvement in patient knowledge.[26] This type of educational method would be useful for pharmacists to assess patients' educational needs while they waited for prescriptions.[26]

Appendix A provides a list of some computer-assisted education available for patients and pharmacists.

Miscellaneous Methods

Other educational methods are available to use in patient counseling. By recording their symptoms in a diary, patients can monitor their progress and determine if the medication is working.

The pharmacist can help the patient to develop a list of questions to ask the physician on his or her next visit. This can help patients to clarify their concerns, as well as improve physician–patient communication, which in turn tends to improve compliance as discussed earlier.

Various patient support groups are often available in the community for conditions such as epilepsy, diabetes, psychiatric problems, and alcohol and drug addiction. Pharmacists should keep a list of such groups and refer patients where appropriate. These types of groups may improve the patient's understanding and attitudes towards his condition and medication use.

Because the family is often an influence on the patient's health attitudes and behavior, family members may also benefit from any of the discussed educational methods as well as involvement in support groups, some specifically geared to patient's families.

A contract (written or verbal) between the pharmacist and patient can also help motivate the patient to comply.

Selection of the Educational Method

Faced with this variety of educational methods for use in counseling, pharmacists may not be sure which to use with their patients. For patient counseling to be most effective, the educational methods used should be appropriate to the context of the learning and the objectives of the learning.[1,27]

The context of the learning depends on the setting, the goals of the patient and the pharmacist, the patient's stage of learning, and the patient's personal style. The objectives of the learning may involve improving the patient's knowledge or his or her understanding of the information provided; developing the patient's skills; or changing the patient's attitude toward medication or illness.

The Context of the Learning

The Setting

The educational methods used by the pharmacist should vary with the setting in which the counseling interaction takes place. The educational methods used may be somewhat limited by the setting for patient counseling, which is often fairly restrictive. Interactions generally occur at the pharmacy counter or in a more private booth or office setting.

In a more private setting, more discussion is possible. In addition, it is easier to provide demonstrations, have the patient practice administering medication, or present audiovisual materials in a private area. Counseling is more effective (in terms of patient knowledge and compliance) when it takes place in a private setting (e.g., in an office adjacent to the waiting area) as opposed to a low-privacy area (e.g., across a counter adjacent to a crowded waiting area).[28] This may be a result not only of the patient's greater ease in a private setting, but also of the approach to counseling that privacy makes possible—one in which the pharmacist and the patient tend to ask more questions and engage in more dialogue.[28]

The lack of complete privacy need not, however, limit the pharmacist to the lecture-style presentation or print information. For example, the pharmacist may be able to find a quiet area in the pharmacy to demonstrate the use of an inhaler, or he may schedule an appointment with the patient at a quieter time, in the pharmacy or at the patient's home. Alternatively, the patient might be allowed to take written or audiovisual materials home and then discuss them later on the telephone with the pharmacist. The telephone is a useful medium for pharmacists to aid in privacy. The setting for patient counseling will be discussed in more detail in Chapter 9.

Goals of the Pharmacist and the Patient

The goals of the pharmacist and the patient should also affect the educational methods selected. The goals of learning may be different from one situation to the next, and any given learning situation may involve several goals.[27] Different teaching methods (or combinations of methods) may be suitable for different learning goals.

For example, one of the counseling goals for a patient receiving a prescription for an inhaler for the first time is to instruct the patient in the proper use of the inhaler. The patient will learn the correct procedure most effectively by observing and imitating a demonstration in the use of the inhaler (modeling), by practicing the procedure repeatedly (rote), and by correcting and altering his or her use of the inhaler in response to failed attempts during practice (trial and error). Alternatively, for a patient receiving a new prescription for an anticoagulant, the pharmacist should explain dosing and the need for continual evaluation through regular blood testing. This patient will learn most effectively by listening to the pharmacist's presentation of the information, and by reading additional print information and discussing it further with the pharmacist.

The pharmacist must identify the specific counseling needs of each patient, and then should select the teaching methods best suited to that purpose.

The Patient's Stage of Learning

Another factor that should affect the educational methods selected is the stage of the patient's learning regarding his or her medication and illness.[27] A patient learning about inhaler use may, at a later stage, have to deal with concerns about using the inhaler around family members or at work. The patient may also have to deal with personal concerns about having to use an inhaler or about the seriousness of his asthmatic condition. These new concerns require a different approach to learning—a more patient-centered approach. The educational method should involve discussion with the patient to help him or her discover where the problems lie and how they may be overcome.

The Patient's Personal Style and Orientation

Many studies in the educational field concern the ways people take in information, make sense of it, and ultimately make use of it, to solve problems, make decisions, and create new meanings.[1] The characteristic ways in which people go through these processes are referred to as cognitive and learning styles.[1]

Cognitive style refers to the manner in which a person organizes experiences into meanings, values, skills, and strategies.[1] Learning style refers to the manner in which a person's meanings, values, skills and strategies undergo change.[1] Learning and cognitive styles are relatively stable traits related to personality structure and are distinct from ability or performance in learning.[1]

Each patient may perceive the goal of the education and the methods used differently, depending on his or her own cognitive and learning styles. For example, some patients may learn more effectively from lectures and reading material, and may actually prefer the medical model approach to the helping approach discussed earlier in Chapter 2.[27] Other patients would prefer the helping approach, with more discussion and interaction with the pharmacist.

The pharmacist must recognize that patients have preferred cognitive and learning styles. Although it would not be practical for the pharmacist to become involved in determining each patient's style, the pharmacist can attempt to accommodate individual preferences by offering a variety of educational methods. As mentioned earlier, patients prefer a combination of counseling methods to one method alone.

Objectives of Learning

Counseling may involve a variety of objectives which will vary with the patient and the situation. Different learning objectives often call for different educational methods, as shown in Table 6.1.

Improving Knowledge

One objective of learning in patient counseling is the improvement of the patient's knowledge regarding his or her medication or illness. To meet this objective, the patient must receive the information and must have the opportunity to internalize it. The most appropriate methods for this purpose involve the provision of information through lectures, dialogue, readings, and audiotapes or videotapes.[29]

Improving Understanding

Another objective of learning in patient counseling is the improvement of the patient's understanding of medication use. Patients may need help in comprehending how their medication can relieve or prevent symptoms and what the implications of their illness or medication use might be with respect to their lifestyles.

The patient must understand how to apply the information provided by the pharmacist. For example, a patient may have the knowledge that alcohol will interact with his or her medication, but may need help in understanding how alcohol use can be curtailed during social or business events. The most appropriate educational methods for this purpose are demonstrations and problem-solving discussions.[29]

Developing Skills

In some patient-counseling situations, one of the objectives of learning is the development of skills, such as using an inhaler. This involves the patient learning through practice. The pharmacist can help the patient to develop new skills by encouraging him or her to practice the required techniques, both in the pharmacy and at home.[29]

Changing Attitudes

Finally, patient counseling may involve the need to change some of the patient's attitudes in order for him or her to get the most benefit from treatment. Patients may need to develop more positive feelings about their medication use or their condition and to become motivated to follow advice. For example, consider a patient who refuses to accept his asthmatic condition and sees no need for regular medication use or modifications in his lifestyle. The objective of learning in this patient's counseling will be the alteration of these attitudes and motivation to change his behavior in regard to treatment.

Such methods as discussion and video simulations may help patients to adopt new attitudes and to become motivated.[29]

Table 6.1   Educational Methods and Learning Objectives

Learning Objective	Most Appropriate Methods
To improve knowledge	*Lecture, dialogue, reading, audio-visual methods*
To improve understanding	*Demonstrations, discussions*
To develop skills	*Encourage the patient to practice techniques*
To change attitudes	*Discussion, video simulations*

Adapted from Knowles, MS. Designing and managing learning activities. In: The Modern Practice of Adult Education: from pedagogy to andragogy. Rev. and Updated, 1980. Cambridge Adult Education. Prentice Hall Regents, Englewood Cliffs, NJ:240.

Counseling one patient can involve all the learning objectives described. Patients must acquire knowledge about their medication and the manner in which it is to be administered; they must understand how the medication is used and how it improves their condition; they must develop skill in administering the medication; and they may need to alter their attitudes about the need for regular medication use. In other words, pharmacists are likely to find that, for maximum effectiveness in patient counseling, they will need to employ a variety of educational methods when counseling patients.

Counseling Aids

In the discussion of noncompliance in Chapter 4, it was suggested that the pharmacist could make use of a variety of counseling aids to assist the patient. Counseling aids such as calendars and various packaging methods may reduce noncompliance by simplifying multiple drug regimens and by helping to overcome difficulties resulting from cognitive or physical impairments.[30]

Currently available counseling aids effectively address noncompliance that arises from difficulties in taking medication, confusion over dosing times, and forgetfulness. However, supplying these counseling aids will not address the many other possible causes of noncompliance.

Medication-Reminder Cards

A medication-reminder card can be prepared on an individual basis by the pharmacist. It may simply consist of a calendar on which each day is divided into sections according to the number of doses to be taken. Patients can mark off each day's squares as they take doses. If more than one medication is used, different markings or colors can be adopted as codes (e.g., an asterisk for one drug and an X for another). The pharmacist can indicate the names of the drugs, the dosing schedule, and any coding used on the calendar.[31] A sample appears in Figure 6.1.

Although some patients may find these useful, Ascione and Shimp found that patients using a medication reminder calendar along with verbal instructions were not more compliant than those receiving only verbal instructions.[32] In addition, patients viewed the calendars negatively, probably because most reported they were already using some sort of reminder system such as keeping drugs in a visible place.[32]

Assisted Labeling

All prescriptions are accompanied by written labels bearing instructions, and auxiliary labels are often added. Some patients, however, may need additional assistance with interpreting or reading labels because of illiteracy, poor vision, or confusion over interpreting or co-ordinating dosing instructions.

As discussed earlier, approximately 40 million Americans are unable to read or have difficulty reading.[16] In addition, many people have vision impairment that hinders reading. In particular, an estimated 20% of the geriatric population suffers from poor eyesight, even with corrective lenses.[1] These data suggest that many patients may be unable to read prescription labels.

Studies of patients' ability to read prescription labels indicate that in addition to reading or vision problems, a high percentage of patients misinterpret prescription-label instructions. In one such study, 73% of the respondents 64 years of age or under and 93% of those 65 years of age or over misinterpreted label instructions such as "Take one on an empty stomach."[33] Confusion also occurred with instructions that involved co-ordinating several different medications with different dosage schedules.[33]

For patients with reading difficulties, the use of a chart with a circular diagram of a 24-hour clock has been suggested, as shown in Figure 6.2.[34] The pharmacist can indicate the number of tablets and the dosage times in the section beside each number on the clock. Color or marking codes could be used to distinguish different types of medications. Patients who have impaired vision might benefit from a medication-instruction clock with embossed dots.[34] A picture of the moon and sun can be added beside "A.M." and "P.M." to further assist nonreaders.

Prescription and auxiliary labels can also be adapted for patients with impaired vision. Some computers can be adapted to provide labels with larger print, and some auxiliary labels are now available with large print, symbols, and Braille.[31]

For patients who find it difficult to interpret instructions or to coordinate the dosing of several different medications, a medication chart may be of assistance (see Figure 6.3). Such a chart would have space for the name of the patient and columns for the name of the medication, the purpose or category of the medication, the dosage instructions, the number of tablets in different columns according to time, and the name of the doctor.[31] This would help patients understand and co-ordinate their complete medication regimen.

Figure 6.1
Medication-Reminder Card

Patient Name:

Month of:

	Sat.	Sun.	Mon.	Tues.	Wed.	Thurs.	Fri.
Name of medication and directions for use							
Name of medication and directions for use							

1. Pharmacist completes name of medication and instructions for use.

2. Patient checks off squares as doses are taken.

Adapted from: Pritchard R, Senders H. Patient compliance aids. On Continuing Practice. 1989;16(3):25-29

Pill-Reminder Containers

Pill-reminder containers assist patients in remembering to take their medications. These containers may be filled by the pharmacist, the patient, a family member, or anyone else involved in the patient's care. They are commercially available, but the pharmacist can also show patients how to devise their own.[31]

Commercially available pill-reminder containers come in a variety of sizes for daily or weekly scheduling. Unfortunately, most only provide one compartment per dosing time, so that several different types of medications must be combined in each container. Another shortcoming of pill-reminder containers commercially available is that some do not include spaces for written instructions to be filled out by the pharmacist.[15]

Figure 6.2
Medication-Instruction Clock

Patient Name:

Medication and Code:

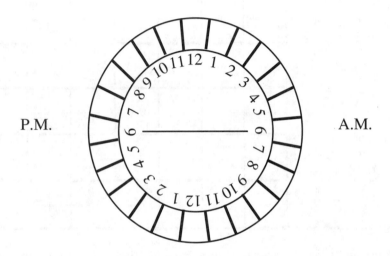

P.M.   A.M.

1. Pharmacist indicates number of tablets in the section beside each number.
2. Pharmacist completes patient name, medication names, and corresponding color or code.

Adapted from: Eustace CA, Johnson GT, Gault MH. Improvements in drug prescription labels for patients with limited education or vision. Can Med Assoc J. 1982;127 (8) :301

Some pill-reminder containers available actually remind patients to take medication by way of an alarm mechanism, while other pill-reminders assist patients by allowing them to keep track of when their medication was taken.[15,35]

Alternatively, patients can make pill-reminder containers out of egg cartons or paper cups that can be filled with medications daily or weekly.

The problem with pill-reminder containers is that they often cannot accommodate complete labelling and they have no child-proofing mechanism. Since pharmacists are required by law to dispense medication with proper labelling, the pharmacist can only make patients aware of pill-reminder containers and possibly have them available for sale in the pharmacy. Patients should be

Figure 6.3
Medication Chart

Patient Name: _____

Medication	Purpose	Dosage	Number of tablets				Doctor
			7 A.M.-9 A.M.	ll A.M.-1 P.M.	4 P.M.-6 P.M.	8 P.M.-10 P.M.	

Pharmacist enters information for each medication.

Adapted from: Pritchard R, Senders H. Patient compliance aids. On Continuing Practice.
1989;16(3):25-29

warned about the lack of child resistance and should be advised to keep their pill-reminder containers out of the reach of children.[31]

The usefulness of these types of counseling aids have been tested. One study found that most patients did not use the pill-reminders, and that patients who were organized already had a system for taking their medication whereas those who were not found the boxes useless.[36] However, another study found that elderly patients provided with counseling in addition to a medication-reminder package reported improved compliance compared to those receiving only counseling or counseling plus a calendar.[32] Patients also believed that the reminder packages were useful.[32]

Unit-of-Use Packaging

Various packaging methods can be used that assist patients by providing one dose of medication at a time, such as blister packaging or individual medication cups.

Medication compliance was found to be significantly better among a group of elderly patients provided with unit-of-use packaging (2-oz plastic cups with snap-on lids containing all drugs to be taken at morning or evening).[36]

Another study used a calendar blister-pack system which provided 31 large blisters on each card.[30] One card was provided for each dosing time (e.g., four cards would be dispensed for 1 month of medication used four times daily).

This packaging resulted in increased compliance over a 3-month study period by a group of ambulatory geriatric clinic outpatients.[30]

Unit-of-use packaging provides a continual intervention that demands little involvement by a health professional once it is set up. It provides reinforcement and cuing, supplies easy instructions, and simplifies medication administration for the patient.[30] There are also a number of disadvantages to some unit-of-use packaging, including inability to add or delete drugs once a pack is set up; minimal flexibility for complex regimens; lack of portability; and higher costs of labor and time in preparation. In addition, some are difficult for certain patients to open, whereas most lack child-resistance.[30]

Dosing Aids

Patients sometimes have difficulty following exact dosing directions because of problems in making accurate measurements. Directions for fractions of tablets or for liquid measurements may be more accurately followed with the help of dosing aids.

Devices that accurately divide tablets of all sizes and shapes are available on the market, as are various pill crushers.[15] Patients should be advised, however, that these devices cannot be used for sustained-release or long-acting medications or for tablets with enteric or protective coating.

Calibrated spoons or various liquid dispensers such as syringes (without needles) are available for administration of liquid medications. This assists in accurate dosing since household teaspoons can range in volume measure from 4 to 7 mL.[31]

Aero-chambers and masks that help direct inhaled medication into the mouth are also available. These assist patients in using inhaled medication whom often fail to get complete doses because they find it difficult to press the inhaler and inhale simultaneously.

Medication Refill Reminder Systems and Telephone Follow-up

As discussed in Chapter 4, increased contact time or supervision by health care professionals can increase medication compliance. This lead to the concept of increasing patient supervision through reminding patients when refills of their medications are due, either by postcards or by telephone calls (either personal or computerized). Follow-up telephone calls to monitor patients also help to increase compliance.

Computerized systems that link to patient records and telephone patients automatically are available. One such system calculates drug usage, determines refill dates, and initiates a telephone call using the actual voice of the pharmacist. It reminds the patient that the drug needs to be refilled, and allows for additional comments by the pharmacist and accepts the patient's response.[15,35]

One study evaluated telephone or postcard refill reminders.[37] A significant increase in compliance occurred in both reminder groups. Interestingly, the control group, who were telephoned to check on their compliance, also improved in compliance after the first month of the study, suggesting that the increase in communication, regardless of whether compliance is encouraged during the conversation, improves compliance.[37] In another study, a follow-up telephone call was made to patients on the fourth or fifth day of therapy to reinforce the importance of compliance and to determine if the patients were having any problems with the prescribed regimen. This intervention was found to increase compliance as effectively as a written and verbal consultation given on the day the medication was dispensed, again possibly because of the increased attention rather than the content alone.[7]

The advantages of such programs include not only their effectiveness in improving compliance, but also their ability to recover the revenue from the 60 to 100 million prescriptions not re-filled each year, approximately $1.6 billion a year. However, the disadvantage can be customer dissatisfaction if the patient has not given permission, as well as the risk to patient confidentiality.[35] One pharmacy chain found that 60% of its customers did not want a phone call or reminder postcard, because they thought it was an invasion of privacy or simply an attempt by the pharmacy to make another sale. This pharmacy chain now uses a brochure to explain the service, and a form for patients to fill out if they prefer a telephone call or a postcard.[35]

Developing Patient-Education Programs in the Pharmacy

The pharmaceutical care process involves identifying real and potential problems, and developing and implementing a plan to overcome these problems.[38] Part of developing the plan often involves developing patient-education programs. Although pharmacists often approach patient-education for all patients in the same way, providing most patients verbal and written counseling, they should develop programs on an individual basis, using the various methods and counseling aids discussed above where appropriate.[39] In addition, pharmacists should develop educational programs for specific groups of patients with similar characteristics, such as the elderly or patients with diabetes.

As part of providing patient education, pharmacists often develop their own educational materials or make presentations. To ensure maximum effectiveness of their efforts, pharmacists should be aware of the educational principles involved in such an endeavor.

Developing an Individual Patient Education Program

Pharmacists can increase the effectiveness of the various educational methods and counseling aids discussed above by going through a planning process that individualizes the education to the patient's needs, abilities, and personal resources.[40] A decision-making process should be used whereby the patient's problems are identified, priorities are established, goals are formulated, appropriate educational intervention is selected, and the intervention is implemented then evaluated (see Table 6.2).[41–43] As discussed in Chapter 5, the counseling process should incorporate these steps.

Table 6.2   Developing an Individual Patient-Education Program

Identify the educational needs of the patient and family

Establish educational goals

Select appropriate educational methods

Implement the educational plan

Evaluate

Adapted from Witte K, Bober K. Developing a patient education program in the community pharmacy. Am Pharm. 1982;NS22(10):28-32.

Identifying the Educational Needs of the Patient and Family

Through the information-gathering and problem-identification stages of the patient-counseling protocol, the pharmacist should evaluate the patient's present knowledge level as well as any problems that require educational intervention. As discussed in Chapters 3 and 4, various factors need to be considered to affect the patient's health behavior. These include the patient's perceptions of severity and risk of his condition; modifying factors such as age, personality, and knowledge; triggers to action such as advice or support from family; and evaluation of perceived benefits against, barriers such as costs and accessibility to care.

The pharmacist should also ask the patient for his own evaluation of his educational needs. Although the family is often not included in this discussion, family members can have a significant influence on the patient's attitudes and behavior and therefore should be considered for inclusion in any educational interventions.

The educational needs identified may involve deficiency in knowledge or understanding, skill, attitudes, or beliefs.

Establishing Educational Goals and Objectives

The goal of the program is the desired outcome stated in a broad way, for example: To provide the patient with information about high blood pressure so he will understand how to self-treat effectively and safely.[41]

Objectives further explain specific behavior that the education should change with respect to knowledge, skills, and attitudes.[41] An objective to change the patient's knowledge may be stated as follows: "By the end of the program the patient will be able to list reasons why medication is needed and state proper dose and times of medication use." An objective to change the patient's attitudes may be stated as: "The patient will believe the consequences of high blood pressure are serious, believe that he can take action to control his blood pressure by complying with medication." An objective to change the patient's skills may be stated as: "The patient will take his medication regularly."

These goals and objectives should be discussed with the patient to be sure that they understand and accept them. In addition, various constraints must be considered so that objectives are realistic. For example, it cannot involve drastic changes in the patient's lifestyle to be accomplished overnight.

Selecting Appropriate Educational Methods

Together with the patient, the pharmacist should consider possible educational options. As discussed above, the selection of the most effective educational methods should take into consideration the objectives as well as the context of learning. In addition to the effectiveness, another more practical consideration will be the efficiency in terms of costs and time for patient and pharmacist.

Implementing the Program

The selected educational methods and materials should be synthesized into a program, and a plan should be made as to when the program should start, how long it will be used, and when it will be assessed.[40,41] The outcomes specified in the objectives should be reviewed and a time agreed on for achieving the objectives and evaluating them. Follow-up should be arranged and carried out.

Evaluating the Program

Plans and methods to evaluate the program should be made early and discussed with the patient. The evaluation should be specific to the goals: for example, if one goal of the program is to change attitude, then some way must be found to ascertain that attitude change has indeed occured. Clearly stated goals and objectives make evaluation easier.

Evaluation should be ongoing, and may involve observing the patient (e.g., using his inhaler); interviewing the patient (during refill counseling or follow-up counseling); asking the patient to complete a questionnaire.

In a study of pharmacists using this systematic process in developing patient education for individual patients, pharmacists spent an average of 81 minutes per patient in the total process.[39] This time included providing a consultation letter to the physician, performing a number of separate patient interactions (patient history, patient assessment, patient education session, feedback telephone call), and planning and documenting. Although the outcomes of the education programs were not evaluated, patient satisfaction was evaluated and found to be very high (averaging 4.4 out of 5 overall).

Developing a Patient-Education Program for Specific Patient Groups

Although patients are all individuals, some similarities in the medication-related problems that they face allow programs to be developed to target specific groups of patients. As discussed above, individual program planning can be time-consuming, and therefore, costly. Some benefits can be accrued in selecting specific patient groups for whom a general educational plan could be developed (e.g., diabetes patients). This plan could then be adapted for use with individual patients.

Pharmacists may select groups of patients who will likely benefit most from education. Examples of such groups include patients on drug therapy with a high iatrogenic potential, such as patients on warfarin or digoxin; and patients for whom compliance is particularly critical, such as those with diabetes or hypertension.[41] Alternatively, pharmacists can select groups of patients who are common among their pharmacy clientele, such as young children or the elderly.

Developing the plan should involve the same elements as for the individual patient, except that the initial step will involve selecting the target group and identifying common problems they may face. Common problems can be identified from reading journal reports, local hospital-admission reports, discussion with other health professionals, or observation during practice as well as from questionnaires conducted within the pharmacy clientele. The patients' perceptions of the need for education should be included with clinical evidence of need, since this will help the pharmacist determine the best way to approach patients for involvement in the program (i.e., there may be a need to overcome initial resistance or raise awareness of problems and the need for education).

When selecting material appropriate to the target population, the pharmacist should select a variety of educational methods so that the program can be easily individualized to the patient's needs. As discussed previously, multiple materials are most effective, and no single strategy is effective for all patients under all circumstances.

Even though the program has been planned for a group, each patient's specific needs should be considered to ensure that his needs will be met by the program. If necessary, changes should be made to the program to accommodate the individual.

Previously Developed Programs for Specific Patient Groups

A variety of education programs developed for specific patient groups have been reported in the literature. Examples of these include programs developed for schizophrenic patients, sight-impaired patients, and the elderly.[35,39,42]

The goals of these programs are varied. A program developed by New York pharmacists for the sight-impaired aimed to improve information provision to patients using prescription labels and communication devices adapted to the needs of the group.[42] The National Council on Patient Information and Education developed a Brown Bag Medicine Review program for the elderly to identify and resolve medication use problems.[35] A Medication Management Module was developed to teach medication self-management skills to schizophrenic patients.[42]

The University of Michigan College of Pharmacy and Institute of Gerontology developed the Focused Drug Therapy Review Program to alter prescriber and patient behavior.[39]

A variety of educational methods were used, including training and skill development, use of specialized prescription labels, one-on-one counseling, oral and written information, medication-reminder packages or calendars, wallet medication cards, and lists of questions to ask the physician.[35,39,42] This is a small sample of the kinds of efforts that can be made by pharmacists today.

Planning an Educational Presentation

As discussed above, presenting various topics about medication use to various groups can be a good educational intervention for pharmacists. It not only provides a good source of information to the public, but also raises the public's awareness of the availability of the pharmacist for individual counseling.

When preparing a presentation, pharmacists need to carefully plan and organize. A series of steps for planning an education presentation are summarized in Table 6.3. The first step involves the pharmacist offering his or her services to local groups.

Table 6.3   Planning an Educational Presentation

Offer services to local groups

Select topics to meet the audience's wants and needs

Gear the information and style of presentation to the audience's level

Be knowledgeable on the topics presented

Use a variety of resources

Organize the speech carefully

Use handout materials, props, audiovisual aids

Involve the audience as much as possible

Ask for feedback

Adapted from Pritchard R. The pharmacist as a public speaker. On Continuing Practice. 1988;15(1)15-18.

Starting small and informally with local community groups or groups of patients gathered in the pharmacy will help the pharmacist to gain confidence. Often the pharmacist is invited to speak by a group, but pharmacists should also contact groups to offer this service. Some potential audiences include senior citizens, women's groups, churches, synagogues, schools, service clubs, special interest groups (e.g., diet groups), drug treatment centers, schools, community centers, and health clubs.[5]

Sometimes the pharmacist is asked to present a particular topic, but it may be left up to the speaker. Suggested presentation topics include safe use of medications, medication for children, nonprescription drugs, drug interactions, drug abuse, or medications for chronic conditions such as diabetes, asthma, hypertension, arthritis, etc.[5] It is important for the pharmacist to be comfortable with the topic and very knowledgeable, although the level of material will vary with the audience. The depth of information, language level, and style of presentation should be adjusted for the expected audience.

Sources of information for talks include journal articles, pharmaceutical companies, and pharmacy organizations. The APhA provides a series of videos along with a planning guide, presentation instructions, audience handouts, and sample news release and promotional items for pharmacists to use in their communities.[2]

When writing the presentation, the old adage "tell them what you're going to tell them, tell them, then tell them what you told them" should be kept in mind. The use of appropriate and tasteful humor as well as props such as examples of medications or pamphlets can add interest, as can audiovisual aids such as slides and videotapes. It is preferable not to read a speech as such, but to speak extemporaneously as much as possible, with a few notecards and props as memory aids.

It is also advisable to involve the audience as much as possible, asking questions and inviting their input. It may be necessary to change the order of topics or to repeat some information to suit the audiences questions.[2] There should be an opportunity for individual audience members to speak with the pharmacist after the presentation, since some people feel uncomfortable asking questions in public. The pharmacist should ask for feedback at the end to help in future presentation planning.[2]

Developing Written Educational Materials

As discussed earlier, written educational materials should be prepared with consideration of the reading level of the general public, and of the specific target audience. One way to ensure this is to test for reading level using a readability formula. This is a mathematical equation that describes the relation between the reader's skill and the author's style of writing to result in a score depicting the level of reading skills needed by the intended reader. A number of tests are available.[44] One such test, the FOG Formula, is one of the easiest methods for calculating grade-level readability. It takes into consideration the structure of the text such as number of words in sentences, total number of words in the text, and the number of syllables in the words (Table 6.4).[44]

Table 6.4 Summary of FOG Readability Index

Count about 100 words. Stop at the nearest sentence end

Count the number of sentences in the 100 words sample (S)

Count the number of hard words (3 syllables or more) (A)

Calculate the grade reading level using the formula

$GL = (100/S + A) \times 0.4$

If the piece is long, repeat this for several 100-word sections and average the results

Adapted from Spadaro D, Robinson L, Smith LT. Assessing readability of patient information materials. Am J Hosp Pharm. 1980;37(2):215-21.

In addition to the difficulty of the words, other aspects of the written material can affect readability. The text organization, including the layout, use of diagrams, charts, colors, or examples, can affect readability as can the reader's background, context clues, reader's interest, and opportunity for reinforcement.[45] When reader interest is high, readability indices may overestimate the difficulty.[45] On the other hand, pain, discomfort, and stress interfere with the patient's concentration and memory, as does the patient's mental state (e.g., possibly confusion, denial, extreme emotions, and hearing or visual disturbances).[45] As a result of these factors, patients forget up to 50% of physicians' statements immediately following their visit.[45]

Certain medical words may not be understood. One reference, "The Living Word Vocabulary: a 43,000 Word Vocabulary Inventory," lists words that were tested for comprehension.[46] Some words such as "void" and "topical" were found to be comprehended by less than 50% of people, and required 12th and 13th grade education level, respectively.[46] The word "drug" had four meanings (medicine, put to sleep, habit forming, and knock out or poison). The authors suggest that the longer word "medication" be used since it generally is taken to mean "healing drug."[46]

Some suggestions for preparing more understandable written information taking the above concerns into consideration, are shown in Table 6.5.

Evaluation of Patient Education Materials

Before embarking on development of materials or programs, pharmacists should check to see what is already available to avoid wasted effort, time, and money. Although pharmacists can develop their own materials, an ever-increasing variety of prepared materials are available as evidenced by the list in Appendix A. However, not all materials are equal, and it is important for pharmacists to evaluate prepared educational materials before using them.

Table 6.5   Suggestions for Preparing Written
Patient-Education Materials

Use short, simple sentences

Use active sentences most of the time (e.g., "swallow each capsule with water")

Use affirmative sentences most of the time unless referring to avoiding an action (e.g., "Take with food," rather than "Do not take on an empty stomach.")

Use common words, preferably one or two syllables, and define medical or technical words. (Use a readability index and adjust to result in Grade 5–6 reading level)

Keep sentences and paragraphs short (10 words or less per sentence)

Introduce one idea per sentence, and limit the number of ideas per page

Be specific (e.g., "Drink at least 8 oz. of water" rather than "Drink plenty of fluid")

Precede information with an advance organizer (e.g., "Things that may reduce back pain are: ...")

Use objectives (e.g., "The following information will help you to use your inhaler")

Use questions followed by information (e.g., "What should I do if I feel dizzy?")

Use headlines and subheadings rather than numbering

Use margins and plenty of empty spaces

Emphasize points with different type face, bold face, underlining, boxing, columns

Use color

Use simple checklists, diagrams, and charts

Use Arabic numbers rather than Roman numerals for letters and lists

Use upper and lower case rather than blocks of capitals which are more difficult to read

Use large print where appropriate such as for the elderly

Adapted from Dolinsky D, Gross S, Deutsch T, et al. Application of psychological principles to the design of written patient information. Am J Hosp Pharm. 1983;40(2):266-71. Hilts L, Krilyk BJ. W.R.I.T.E. Write readable information to educate. Chedoke-McMaster Hospital, Hamilton Civic Hospitals, Hamilton General Division, 1989.

The same principles that apply to preparing written materials apply to evaluating existing written materials. Criteria for selecting patient-education videos have been suggested by Blouch as follows:[47]

1. Uses a vocabulary that is not above the reading level of your patient;
2. Has graphics to help simplify complex medical terminology;
3. Presents the information concisely and in an appropriate sequence so progressive patient learning can be accomplished;
4. Contains practical information appropriate for the individual patient;
5. Displays high-quality audio and visual clarity; and
6. Is no more than 10 minutes long in order to maintain the patient's attention.

Additional considerations in selecting materials are cost and availability.

Materials that do not adhere to the above standards do not necessarily need to be rejected. Since it is advisable to use written or audiovisual materials in conjunction with verbal counseling, any shortfalls can be overcome through discussion with the patient to identify misunderstandings, and verbal reinforcement can be provided. If materials are to be viewed or read by the patient at home, the pharmacist should be sure to follow-up (in person or by telephone) to answer any questions or concerns raised by the material.

Summary

Pharmacists have many resources available provided they are prepared to retrieve them and take the initiative to use them. Studies show that no single strategy is effective for all patients under all circumstances.[48] In addition, patients' attitudes towards pharmacists have been found to be more positive when any information was provided, regardless of the method used.[49] Many of the educational methods and counseling aids discussed in this chapter were found to be more effective when verbal counseling was a component of patient education. Thus, pharmacists need to be good communicators to be effective in verbal counseling. This will be discussed in the following chapter.

References

1. Brundage DH, MacKeracher D. Characteristics of the Adult Learner. Adult Learning Principles and Their Application to Program Planning. Toronto: Ontario Ministry of Education, Ontario Institute for Studies in Education. 1980.

2. Nelson M. Our guest for tonight is...Pharmacists and public speaking. Am Pharm. 1993;NS33(3);59-62.

3. McKay M, Davis M, Fanning P. Public speaking. In: Messages: The Communication Book, Oakland, CA: New Harbinger Publications. 1983.

4. Gondin W, Mamman E. The art of speaking made simple. Rev. Ed. : Garden City, New York: Doubleday & Co., 1981.

5. Pritchard, R. The pharmacist as a public speaker. On Continuing Practice.1988;15(1):15-18.

6. Anon. U.S. Indian services to rethink Rx counseling. Drug Store News for the Pharmacist. 1991;1(5);21.

7. Garnett W, Davis L, McKenney J, et al. Effect of telephone follow-up on medication compliance. Am J Hosp Pharm. 1981;38(5):676-679.

8. Feegel K, Dix Smith M. Counseling and cognitive services for Medicaid patients under OBRA-'90. Pharm Times. 1992;9 Supp:1-9.

9. McBean BJ, Blackburn JL. An evaluation of four methods of pharmacist-conducted patient education. Can Pharm J. 1982;115:167-172.

10. Mullen PD, Gren LW. Measuring patient drug information transfer: An assessment of the literature. Washington, DC: Pharmaceutical Manufacturers Association, 1984.

11. Chermak G, Jinks M. Counseling the hearing-impaired older adult. Drug Intell Clin Pharm.1981;15(5):377-382.

12. Harvey J, Plumridge RJ. Comparative attitudes to verbal and written medication information among hospital outpatients. DICP. 1991;25(9):925-928.

13. Culbertson V, Arthur T, Rhodes P, et al. Consumer preferences for verbal and written medication information. Drug Intell Clin Pharm.1988;22(5):390-396.

14. Cataldo R. OBRA-'90 and your pharmacy computer system. Am Pharm.1992;NS32(11):39-41.

15. Anon. Resources showcase. Talk about prescriptions month. Planning guide. Washington, DC: National Council on Patient Information and Education. October, 1992.

16. Powers R. Emergency department patient literacy and the readability of patient-directed materials. Ann Emerg Med. 1988;17(2):124-126.

17. Work D. We've come a long way...or have we? Am Pharm. 1987;NS27(7):496-498.

18. Marshall WR, Rothenberger MA, Bunnell SL. The efficacy of personalized audiovisual patient-education materials. J Fam Pract 1984;19(5): 659-663.

19. McElnay JC., Scott MG, Armstrong AP, et al. Use of video for patient counseling. Pharm J. 1988; 241(Supp 6508):R28.
20. Olsenk MS, Du Bé JE. Evaluation of two methods of patient education. Am J Hosp Pharm. 1985;42(3):622-624.
21. Soflin D, Young WW, Clayton BD. Development and evaluation of an individualized patient education program about digoxin. Am J Hosp Pharm. 1977;34(4):367-371.
22. Darr MS, Self TH, Ryan MR, et al. Content and retention evaluation of an audiovisual patient education program on bronchodilators. Am J Hosp Pharm. 1981;38(5):672-675.
23. Putnam GL, Yanagisako K. Skin cancer comic book: evaluation of a public educational vehicle. J Audiovisual Media Med. 1985;8(1):22-25.
24. Mahoney C, Jeffrey L, Powlina A. Recorded medication messages for ambulatory patients. Am J Hosp Pharm. 1983;40(3):448-449.
25. Ascione F, Fish C. Computer health/medication information software-compilation for pharmacists. Am Pharm. 1986;NS26(2):45-50.
26. Beck R, Ellis L, Scott D, et al. Microcomputer as patient education. Am J Hosp Pharm. 1982;39(12):2105-2108.
27. Simpson EL. Adult learning theory: A state of the art. In: Adult Development and Approaches to Learning, ed. Moore J, Lasker H, Simpson E. US Government Document: Washington, DC. Sept 1980.
28. Beardsley R, Johnson C, Wise G. Privacy as a factor in patient counseling. J Am Pharm Assoc.1977;17(6):366-368.
29. Knowles MS. Designing and managing learning activities. In: The Modern Practice of Adult Education: From Pedagogy to Andragogy. Englewood Cliffs, NJ: Prentice Hall Regents, 1980.
30. Wong B, Norman D. Evaluation of a novel medication aid, the calendar blister-pak and its effect on drug compliance in a geriatric outpatient clinic. J Am Ger Soc. 1987;35(1):21-26.
31. Pritchard R, Senders H. Patient compliance aids. On Continuing Practice.1989;16(3): 25-29.
32. Ascione F, Shimp L. The effect of four educational strategies in the elderly. Drug Intell Clin Pharm. 1984;18(11):926-931.
33. Hurd P, Butkovich L. Compliance problems and the older patient: Assessing functional limitations. Drug Intell Clin Pharm. 1986;20(3): 228-230.
34. Eustace CA, Johnson GT, Gault MH. Improvements in drug prescription labels for patients with limited education or vision. Can Med Assoc J.1982;127(8):301.
35. Clepper I. Noncompliance the invisible epidemic. Drug Topics. 1992;136(16):44-50,56-65.
36. Cramer J. Compliance: Uncovering the hidden problems in practice. Drug Topics.1992;Supp 136(13):6-10.

37. Murray M, Birt J, Manatunga A, et al. Medication compliance in elderly outpatients using twice-daily dosing and unit-of-use packaging. Ann Pharmacother. 1993;27(5):616-621.
38. Strand LM, Cipolle R, Morley P. Pharmaceutical care: an introduction. Current Concepts. The Upjohn Company, Kalamazoo, Michigan 1992:15.
39. Opdycke RA, Ascione F, Shimp L, et al. A systematic approach to educating elderly patients about their medications. Pat Educ Couns. 1992;19:43-60.
40. Strodtman LA. Decision-making process for planning patient education. Pat Educ Couns. 1984;5(4):189-200.
41. Witte K, Bober K. Developing a patient education program in the community pharmacy. Am Pharm.1982;NS22(10):28-32.
42. Bond W, Hussar D. Detection methods and strategies for improving medication compliance. AJHP. 1991;48(9):1978-1988.
43. Stratton T, Foster P. The British Columbia seniors' brown bag clinic pilot project: Medication problems identification and participant assessments. Can J Aging. 1992;11(2):150-168.
44. Spadaro D, Robinson L, Smith LT. Assessing readability of patient information materials. Am J Hosp Pharm.1980;37(2):215-221.
45. Hilts L, Krilyk BJ. W.R.I.T.E. Write readable information to educate. Hamilton, Ontario, Canada: Chedoke-McMaster Hospital, Hamilton Civic Hospitals, Hamilton Geriatric Division. 1989.
46. Wilson J, Hogan L. Readability testing of auxiliary labels. Drug Intell Clin Pharm.1983;17(1):54-55.
47. Blouch, D. Tuning into patient videos. Pharm Pract. 1993;9(4):38.
48. Anon. Researcher calls Rx package inserts ineffective. Drug Store News.1984;6(22):62.
49. Kimberlin C, Berardo D. A comparison of patient education methods used in community pharmacies. J Pharm Market Manag.1987;1(4):75-94.

7
COMMUNICATION SKILLS IN PATIENT COUNSELING

Counseling as a Communication Challenge

"Communication" has become a buzzword for health professionals in recent years. This focus on patient–health professional communication grew out of concern over patient noncompliance with therapeutic regimens.[1] As discussed in Chapter 4, many investigations undertaken into noncompliance resulted in conflicting information, but one important finding was that providing information alone does not necessarily improve compliance, particularly over the long term. Information is only useful to patients if they notice, understand, and remember it.[2] Investigations involving patient–health professional communications suggested that effective communication may be the key to accomplishing this and therefore improving patient care.[3]

As discussed in Chapter 2, counseling is a helping process. As such, it requires the pharmacist to help the individual to describe his situation and real or potential problems with medication use; it requires the pharmacist to listen well enough to grasp the meaning of what the patient is saying and therefore identify problems; and it requires the pharmacist to discuss the resolution of problems in a way that is understandable and acceptable to the patient.[4] To accomplish this the pharmacist must be able to communicate with the patient effectively.

Many pharmacists believe that people are inherently good or bad communicators and that they cannot be taught to communicate; however, communication is indeed a learned ability.[5] Theories and techniques of communication have been developed, and specific communication skills have been identified. When pharmacists are taught communication skills, improvements are evident in their counseling.[6] Effective patient–pharmacist communication is a critical element in patient counseling.

Since patient counseling often involves contact with other health professionals, pharmacists also need skills in communicating with other members of the health-care team. In the course of providing pharmaceutical care, pharmacists need to be able to communicate effectively with physicians and nurses in order to gather more detailed information about the patient and to discuss the patient's medication problems.

Pharmacists also need to be able to communicate effectively with other pharmacists and pharmacy personnel, both within their own organization and others. Within the pharmacy, pharmacists must work co-operatively together with other pharmacists and pharmacy personnel for the benefit of the patient. Hospital and community pharmacists need to be able to discuss a patient's discharge medications.

The aim of communication training for pharmacists should be to raise the individual's awareness of communication skills and to help identify and enhance existing skills and attitudes to communication.[5] This chapter will present an overview of what communication entails in order to raise awareness of communication with respect to patient counseling. Specific communication and interviewing skills will be discussed, as will communication with other health professionals and pharmacy personnel. A listing of the many available journal articles and books regarding communication is provided in Appendix A for further reading.

As discussed in Chapter 6, various forms of communication can be used during patient counseling and education including speeches, lectures, small-group presentations, and one-to-one discussion. This chapter, however, concerns only one-to-one discussion, which may involve verbal communication (in person and by telephone), nonverbal communication, and written communication.

Understanding Communication

As a basis for understanding communication in pharmacy, and the skills used in patient counseling, a number of communication and counseling theories have been put forth. These theories provide insight into communication as an exchange of messages, psychological aspects, the interactionist approach, and consideration of human needs and values.

Communication as an Exchange of Messages

One way to view communication is as a process in which information is exchanged between two individuals (the pharmacist and the patient in the case of patient counseling).[7] An idea (message) is formed in the mind of the sender and is translated into a form that can be transmitted by spoken or written words or by body language (e.g., an extended hand to greet a person). The message is transmitted by the (pharmacist), perceived by the receiver (patient) through hearing or seeing, and then translated to determine the meaning of the message (e.g., the extended hand was a greeting).

Unfortunately, the message translated by the receiver is often not identical to that transmitted by the sender, and the result is a misunderstanding between the pharmacist and patient. This is apparent through a feedback message provided by the patient as to how the message was perceived and translated. The pharmacist must be alert to this feedback and be prepared to modify and clarify the message as necessary.[8] There may be a number of barriers to communication that can distort the message or inhibit feedback.[7] Such barriers will be discussed further in Chapter 9.

Psychological Theories

Communication is further complicated by the complexities of individual personalities. Various psychological types have been described to help explain how people interact.[9] Although this may appear to stereotype people, it does acknowledge that even though no two people are totally alike, there are identifiable similarities in each of us. These commonalities are seen as pairs of opposing aspects of personality that describe a person's preferences with respect to interest in the outer world, perception, decison making, and approach to life.[9]

The two extremes of attitude towards life are extroversion and introversion. Extroverted behavior involves turning outward to act, looking forward to socializing, being energized by people and events. Introverted behavior involves turning inward, being energized more by inward reflection rather than by socializing.[9]

People also have different perception styles that affect how they take in information through sensing or intuition. Sensing involves being systematic and detail conscious, able to see the big picture. The other extreme is intuition, which involves using insights and hunches rather than concrete details.[9]

People also vary by the way that they make decisions about information ranging from thinking to feeling. Those who use thinking to make decisions tend to be objective, considering causes and outcomes in an impersonal manner. Conversely people who use feeling to make decisions are more likely to be subjective and personal, weighing the values of choices and how others may be affected.[9]

People tend to approach life in different ways, tending to rely mainly on judgment or perception. Those who rely on judgment aim to control events and live in a decisive and planned way. Those who rely more on perception tend to be more spontaneous and flexible, aiming to understand and adapt to life rather than to control it.[9]

Although people can generally identify themselves within a continuum between these sets of opposite psychological types, one end is no better than the other, it simply helps us to see a different perspective in the way people communicate.

The personality traits of both pharmacist and patient will be involved in communication. Although the pharmacist cannot know the personality of each patient, the pharmacist can recognize that it will affect interactions. Also, although these traits are fairly stable, the pharmacist can modify his or her own behavior to become more effective in communicating: for example, to be slightly less extroverted, or to use a little more intuition during patient counseling.

One study considered pharmacists' personality types as it related to nonprescription counseling.[10] Patients counseled by pharmacists who were more extroverted were less likely to change their purchase decision. The authors suggested that the patients may have perceived these pharmacists as unreliable and untrustworthy.

Transactional Analysis Theory

The transactional analysis (TA) theory further helps us to understand the way people interact during counseling. Eric Berne observed that everyone's personality consists of three distinct ego states that describe consistent patterns of feeling, experiencing, and behaving: the parent, adult and child.[7,11] People of all ages can react in these ego states, and Berne suggests that during communication, a transaction occurs between people's ego states.

The parent state incorporates attitudes and behavior taught by an individual's parents and often causes people to respond automatically in the manner their parents or other authority figures would have (nurturing or critical).[7] The child ego state contains the feelings an individual had as a child, and tends to emerge with an emotional response, often in response to another person's parent state (either free and irresponsible or adapted and obedient).[7] The adult ego state causes people to respond more analytically, gathering information, reasoning out a decision, or predicting consequences of actions.[7] It is less automatic than the parent or child states.

Generally, the ideal is for both parties in an interaction to be communicating in the adult state. Sometimes, people have a preferred ego state or find that they react in particular ego states in certain kinds of situations. Also, communication between two people often involves unconscious and destructive ways of relating (games). Health-care professionals often use the parent ego state, and as a result, patients often respond in the child state (free or adapted), or critical parent, resulting in problems in communication.

> Example:
> Pharmacist (parent ego): You must take these pills, or you'll have a heart attack.
> Patient (adapted child ego): Yes alright.
> > Or (free child ego): I don't want to take those horrible pills, and you can't make me.
> > Or (critical parent ego): You can't tell me what to do. Of course I'm not going to have a heart attack.

None of these are desired responses, since they either create friction or encourage dependence by the patient rather than self-responsibility. The desired transaction is "adult" to "adult."

> Example:
> Pharmacist (adult ego): It would be in your best interest if you followed the instructions carefully for this heart medication for the reasons I've explained.
> Patient (adult ego): Yes I understand that. I'll do my best to take them as you suggested.

This approach to understanding communication has been used in the health care field, particularly with respect to solving problems and in encouraging self-responsibility by the patient.[12]

Human Needs

All humans have the same basic needs, and these needs motivate a person's behavior.[7] These five basic needs as described by the psychologist Abraham Maslow include: 1) physiological needs (to eat, sleep, breathe, avoid pain, etc.); 2) safety needs (to be free from physical harm); 3) belonging needs (to be loved and to belong); 4) esteem needs (to feel good about oneself, independence, achievement); 5) self-actualization (to creatively fulfil your potential).[7] This is a hierarchy, so that physiological needs must be met before an individual will be concerned with safety, and so forth. People strive to satisfy these needs, so that when a need is perceived (e.g., hunger), an individual's goal will be to satisfy that need.

During communication each individual will be attempting to satisfy his needs. For example, a patient's attempt to satisfy physiological needs might cause him to ask for his analgesic prescription in a hurry to relieve his pain; while the pharmacist's need for esteem and self-actualization (fulfilling his or her potential as a health professional) will cause him or her to try to discuss the medication with the patient regardless of this pain. The result may be frustration for both parties, unless the pharmacist recognizes the patient's needs and attempts to find a way to satisfy both of their needs.

Individual Values

Individuals have preferences for certain activities, characteristics, or ways of being and for a particular way of life—these are their values.[7] For example, a pharmacist may have chosen to be a pharmacy owner because he likes to be independent, likes status in his community, wants to help others who are ill, and has a duty to his father to take over the business.

As with an individual's needs, the patient and pharmacist may have different values that affect communication. For example, the pharmacist may value authority and want to dictate to the patient regarding compliance; but the patient may value independence and want to take his medication in his own way. The opposing values will lead to conflict in any communication between the patient and pharmacist.

Although people's values do not change readily, pharmacists can at least become aware of their own values and how they may affect their communication. As well, pharmacists should be aware that others may have different values than theirs, and respect those values.[7] This awareness of values will serve to improve communication.

Model of Communication in Pharmacy

The result of considering these models and theories is a complicated picture of communication. In formulating and transmitting a message to the patient, the pharmacist must consider the values, needs, psychological type, and ego state of both himself or herself and his or her patient, and he must consider these factors when interpreting the feedback from the patient. In addition, the pharmacist should recognize that these psychological factors as well as various environmental factors can act as barriers to the transmission and feedback of the message.

Pharmacists certainly aren't going to psychoanalyze everyone they deal with; however, they can use their understanding of the communication models to realize that the patients they deal with may be very different from each other and different from the pharmacists themselves. Pharmacists should therefore be prepared to modify and adjust their messages to suit each patient. Finding ways to modify and adjust the message is the essence of communication skills.

Conditions for Effective Communication in Pharmacy

In order for pharmacists to communicate effectively with patients, a number of conditions need to be met. These conditions involve the pharmacist's approach to the interaction and the atmosphere set by the pharmacist. Pharmacists can provide the appropriate conditions by establishing a helping and trusting pharmacist–patient relationship, demonstrating empathy towards patients, attending to nonverbal communication, being assertive, arranging for privacy, and displaying a degree of emotional objectivity.[13] The techniques involved in doing this will be described in the following pages.

Establishing a Helping Relationship

To understand the value of establishing a helping relationship, consider the following situation.

Counseling Situation

Patty Lester is a 24-year-old woman. Her patient profile indicates that she has received several prescriptions from a certain pharmacy over the past few months. Another pharmacist also practicing at the pharmacy apparently conducted her medication history, and was on duty when her previous prescriptions were filled. Although this pharmacist had seen her in the pharmacy looking around in the nonprescription medication aisle just a few days ago, he had not yet had the opportunity to speak with her. Her medication history indicates that she had received sulfisoxazole tablets for a urinary tract infection several years ago. Today she brings in a prescription for Bactrim DS[R] tablets.

Pharmacist: OK Ms. Lester, your prescription is ready for you.

Patient: (*stooped shoulders, hanging head, flat voice*) Thanks.

Pharmacist: This is an antibacterial tablet to treat your urinary tract infection. Take 1 tablet every 12 hours until they're all gone.

Patient: (*looking doubtful*) OK.

Pharmacist: (*noticing her doubt*) It's just the usual dose. Be sure to take the pills with plenty of water and take them on an empty stomach.

Patient: (*nods her head*)

Pharmacist: (*handing her a patient information leaflet*) Here's some more information about them. (*points to various sections on the leaflet and reviews the information about adverse effects*) They might also make you more sensitive to the sun, so stay out of the sun or wear a sunscreen.

Patient: (*in a depressed voice*) I don't think I'll be doing any sunning.

Pharmacist: Fine. Here's your medication then. Do you have any questions?

Patient: No, I guess not.

Pharmacist: OK. Goodbye then.

Discussion

The nonresponsiveness of this patient made it difficult for the pharmacist to deal with the situation properly. Although he gave the patient all the correct information, he did not gather sufficient information to identify real or potential medication-related problems. In addition, he did not attempt to explore her apparently depressed state or her doubtfulness. In fact, she wasn't feeling at all well and was depressed because the medication instructions would interfere with her plans for a weekend away. She was intending to take the medication, as she had taken a previous sulfisoxazole prescription, two tablets twice daily because she wanted to get better fast. She was also worried about having another urinary tract infection and the implications of this for future child-bearing.

This scenario illustrates the importance of the pharmacist establishing a helping relationship with the patient.

Establishing a helping and trusting relationship involves becoming familiar with the patient, establishing a feeling of trust, and making the patient feel sufficiently comfortable to discuss personal matters and to express herself.[13] This in turn leads to a cooperative and harmonious interaction.[13] This is also referred to by some as developing a "rapport."[14]

Research has shown that when a trusting relationship is established between patients and their health professionals, patients recover more quickly, experience less pain, and experience a greater variety of physiological, psychological, and behavioral gains than do patients who do not have this relationship.[15]

Although a helping and trusting relationship with a patient may develop over time through an ongoing process, it is necessary to establish some degree of a relationship during the initial interaction.

Establishing a helping relationship involves a number of elements (see Table 7.1). The friendly atmosphere of the patient–pharmacist interaction helps to develop a helping relationship. The pharmacist should begin each patient-counseling encounter by greeting the patient by name, introducing himself or herself to the patient, and spending a few minutes in general conversation (e.g., discussing the weather, news, family, etc.).[13] This initial "small talk," however, should be kept relatively brief since the patient will probably be anxious to discuss the matter at hand, as well as for practicality.[13]

A friendly interaction may occur whenever the pharmacist comes in contact with a patient, even if the patient is just asking the location of a particular product in the pharmacy. The pharmacist who goes out of his or her way to talk with and become familiar with a patient (regardless of the topic) has started to develop a helping relationship. Future encounters with the patient for medication counseling will likely be more effective as a result of such seemingly unimportant interactions.

Establishing a helping relationship also involves the actual content of the interaction, which must reflect the pharmacist's genuine interest in and concern for the patient.[15] With a new patient, the time that the pharmacist devotes to the patient during the medication-history interview and the explanation that patient records are maintained for the patient's benefit will convey interest and concern. During prescription or nonprescription counseling, the pharmacist further develops a helping relationship by inviting questions. Responses to patients' questions need to be considered carefully to ensure that the patient's real needs are being met.

During counseling, the pharmacist <u>
to the patient's concerns. The pharmacist'<u>
will assist in establishing a helping rela<u>

The pharmacist's nonverbal langu<u>
and empathy for the patient. Recognitic<u>
assist the pharmacist in identifying a<u>

140 / Pharmacists Talkin

Patient: She
four times
Pharma
only
Pati

Table 7.1 Ways to Esta

- *Greeting: Friendly and unhurri*
- *Conversation: Brief general conversation*
- *Personal Attention: Introduce self and use patient's name*
- *Invite requests and respond to questions appropriately*
- *Demonstrate Genuine Interest and Concern: Spend time, explain, display empathy*
- *Nonverbal language: Showing attentiveness, interest and concern*

Alternate Counseling Situation

Although the pharmacist had not counseled Patty for a prescription before, he had seen her in the pharmacy just a few days ago. He took the opportunity to speak with her by asking if she needed any help. This resulted in a consultation for a sunscreen product that Patty was purchasing. Today when she brings in a prescription for Bactrim DS[R] tablets, the pharmacist reminds her of this.

Pharmacist: OK Patty, your prescription is ready for you. Come into the booth over here where we can speak more privately.

Patient: *(stooped shoulders, hanging head, flat voice)* Thanks.

Pharmacist: I remember speaking with you a few days ago about a sunscreen for your holiday weekend coming up. That lake you were telling me about sounded like a great place. But you look a little down today.

Patient: *(sounding depressed)* This bladder infection is making me feel so lousy.

Pharmacist: Yes, bladder infections can be pretty uncomfortable. It's a good thing you've got that holiday weekend coming up so you can have a good rest.

Patient: *(brightening a little)* I don't know if I'll be able to go. I hope these pills work fast.

Pharmacist: These pills should start making you feel better within 2 to 3 days. I would like to spend a few minutes going over some information to make sure you get the most benefit from them. *(pause)*

Patient: Yes, alright.

Pharmacist: How did the doctor tell you to take them?

...dn't say much. I guess it's the same as last time, two tablets a day.

...st: Well actually, these are a little different from last time. You ...ed to take one tablet twice daily.

...ent: *(looking doubtful and thinks she might take them four times a day ...yway so they'll work faster)* OK.

Pharmacist: *(noticing her doubt)* You look a little doubtful. These will work just as well, probably better than the other ones. You just don't need so many pills.

Patient: Oh really? I guess two a day will be easier to remember anyway. *(decides to take only two daily as directed)*

Pharmacist: *(hands her a patient-information leaflet)* Here's some more information about how to take them. *(points to various sections on the leaflet and reviews the information about scheduling dosing and drinking fluid)* Do you think you'll be able to stick to a schedule while you're away?

Patient: I think so. I'll make a note on my calendar and in my day-timer.

Pharmacist: Good idea. It's important to take them regularly and to finish them right up, to make sure the infection is completely gone.

Patient: I'll be sure to take them all. I don't want this to go on any longer than it has to.

Pharmacist: Good. Now I need to tell you more information. Occasionally, unwanted effects occur with this medication, although they're unlikely to happen to you, it's best if you are aware of what to notice. *(mentions those noted on the information sheet)* If you notice any of these symptoms, let me know right away.

Patient: OK.

Pharmacist: It also mentions here that this may make you more sensitive to the sun. Be sure to wear that sunscreen you bought the other day.

Patient: Yes, I always wear sunscreen.

Pharmacist: I noticed the doctor has just ordered one course of the medication for you. Did she arrange to see you again?

Patient: No, she just said to come back if the symptoms come back again.

Pharmacist: Fine. Do you have any questions about this?

Patient: Well, I was wondering about having so many bladder infections. Do you think it will affect my being able to have a baby?

Pharmacist: *(proceeds to discuss the patient's concerns, providing information about bladder infections and ways to prevent infections, and encouraging her to discuss the details of her condition and her concerns further with her physician, then closes the discussion)* Here's your prescription then. I hope you're feeling better soon. Give me a call before you go away to let me know how it's going.

Patient: *(smiling)* OK, I'll do that. It sounds like I'll be feeling well enough to go after all. Thanks for everything. Goodbye.

Discussion

This time the pharmacist had laid the groundwork for medication counseling by interacting with the patient on a previous occasion. He tried to make her feel relaxed and comfortable in the counseling session by introducing himself and discussing her vacation. The pharmacist observed the patient's nonverbal language, noticing that she was not her usual self. He demonstrated genuine interest and concern in the patient, allowing her to feel comfortable disclosing her concern about not being well enough to go away for the weekend and her intention to be noncompliant. By inviting questions from the patient, the pharmacist further showed his willingness to listen, opening up the discussion to more important concerns the patient had about her condition. To further establish the relationship, the pharmacist arranged to follow-up with the patient later in the week.

Demonstrating Empathy Towards the Patient

Patient care is often provided in a distant, impersonal manner, and many patients feel that the health care professionals don't really care or understand their questions or concerns.[16] Since the theories discussed above suggest that much of communication involves an individual's feelings and beliefs, pharmacists need to find ways to recognize these aspects of the patient and respond to them. This is the essence of demonstrating empathy.

Patient counseling is essentially based on empathy. When the pharmacist demonstrates empathy towards the patient, the patient sees the pharmacist's interest and concern. This improves the patient's sense of worth and dignity, which may have been temporarily diminished as a result of illness. The patient feels encouraged to voice concerns and problems (or anticipated problems) regarding his illness or medication use. The pharmacist is then better able to assess accurately the patient's needs, concerns, motivations, and level of knowledge in order to provide the appropriate information and reassurance.[17] Thus, the pharmacist who can feel and demonstrate empathy for the patient will be an effective patient counselor.

What is Empathy?

Consider the following situation:

A pharmacist is working in a community pharmacy on a very busy afternoon. He is, as usual, trying to do several things at once, and the pharmacy technician is away for the afternoon. The pharmacist is preparing prescriptions for several waiting patients, but is continually interrupted by telephone calls. He has just taken a prescription over the phone from a dentist, Dr. Jordan. As he puts down the phone, a patient starts banging on the counter and yelling, in a loud and angry voice, "Can't someone help me here? I'm in a hurry and I have to pick up the prescription that Dr. Jordan phoned in for me."

The pharmacist turns quickly toward the patient with a surprised expression, and accidentally knocks over a bottle of antibiotic liquid. He cries out, "Oh no!" and leans on the counter with his hands over his face, shaking his head.

If you can imagine what the pharmacist is feeling at that moment—his emotions, his concerns, his frustrations—then you are feeling empathy. Empathy involves understanding the world as another person sees it, attempting to "get into his shoes."[9] It is the ability to understand not only the other person's words but also what those words mean in terms of his feelings.[17] Demonstrating empathy involves communicating this understanding. In order to do this, you must first be able to identify the person's feelings and meanings then communicate this understanding by responding empathetically.

Identifying Feelings and Meanings

In the scenario described, it may have been easy for the reader to empathize with the pharmacist, because most people have experienced spilling something before. Empathizing with the patient may be more difficult for the reader and for the pharmacist in the scenario. Close observation of the patient, the expression on his face, and other manifestations of nonverbal language, may help to tell the pharmacist more about the patient's emotion.

Another clue to identifying feelings is to imagine the range of emotions the patient might be experiencing and to try to isolate the one that predominates. The patient who says he is "in a hurry" may be feeling worried, frustrated, or in pain.

The pharmacist must also interpret the patient's words to identify their true meaning.[18] Is the patient saying that he is in a hurry because he is in pain, because he feels he is wasting his time treating an unimportant condition, or simply because he has an appointment to go to? One way to help identify the patient's feelings is for the pharmacist to ask himself, "What one word describes the patient's feeling when he made that statement?"[19] In the scenario, the word may be "anger" or "frustration." That one word or a variation of it can be used in an empathetic response to the patient.

Responding Empathetically

The pharmacist must communicate to the patient, in a nonjudgmental way, that he understands and accepts the patient's feelings and concerns, even if those feelings make the pharmacist feel uncomfortable.[17] The pharmacist must verbally encourage the patient to express concerns and feelings, while conveying an attitude of concern and acceptance.[17,18] This recognition and acceptance helps the patient to become less anxious and more open to discussion of his or her problems.[18]

Pharmacists often have difficulty formulating an empathetic response. Sometimes we say, "Yes, I understand how you must feel," and then receive the angry and frustrated retort, "No, you don't! How could you possibly understand?"

In a more complete response, active listening, the pharmacist would reflect the patient's feeling, then paraphrase the patient's comments to include a possible reason for the feelings. For example, "You sound pretty angry about having to wait here so long."

The pharmacist may not be sure about the accuracy of his interpretations, and should ask the patient for clarification: "Is it because you're in so much pain?"

If the pharmacist happens to misinterpret the patient's feelings or meaning, the patient can correct him, but he will nonetheless have received the message that the pharmacist is interested and concerned.[19] The patient may reply, "I'm in pain, and the dentist didn't even help. He says he can't do anything today until I get rid of the infection."

Empathetic responding may be used alone or in combination in a discussion with a patient, until the patient's emotional state has been resolved.[20]

A formula for an active listening response includes a "feeling reflection" and a "content reflection" as follows:

"You feel_____because_____."[15] It also helps to vary the introductory phrase such as:[19]

"You think..."

"It seems to you..."

"As I understand it, you seem to be saying..."

"You believe..."

"In other words..."

"I gather that..."

As an illustration of the value of demonstrating empathy in counseling, consider the following.

Counseling Situation

Mrs. Miller has adult-onset diabetes which had been controlled through diet alone until recently. She has undergone testing and has just come from her physician with a new prescription for glyburide 5 mg, one tablet daily. She is a regular customer at this pharmacy and the pharmacist Alison knows her fairly well. When the prescription is prepared she calls Mrs. Miller into the counseling booth.

Pharmacist: Hello, Mrs. Miller. How are you today?

Patient: *(in a subdued voice)* Oh, I'm OK, I guess.

Pharmacist: I'll just spend a few minutes to discuss your prescription with you to make sure you get the most benefit from it.

Patient: *(looking distracted)* OK.

Pharmacist: This medication is glyburide. What did the doctor tell you about it?

Patient: *(sounding worried)* She told me that the diet I was on for my sugar isn't working, and so I have to take pills now. She says I'm a diabetic, and I know that's really bad. My friend has a son who had all kinds of problems with it.

Pharmacist: Don't worry, Mrs. Miller. Lots of people have diabetes at your age. It's nothing to worry about. As long as you take your pills regularly, you'll be just fine. You must take one tablet every day. You should be testing your blood sugar regularly to check that the pills are working. Here's an information sheet listing the signs of low blood sugar *(refers to a written list)* and here's a list of side effects. *(again refers to written information)*

Patient: *(cutting in, visibly distressed)* All this and side effects too?

Pharmacist: Yes, but don't worry. They don't happen very often. By the way, you shouldn't drink alcohol because it may make you sick. Do you see any difficulties with following these instructions?

Patient: *(stunned into silence, simply shakes her head)*

Pharmacist: Good. Do you have any questions?

Patient: *(in a shaky voice)* No, I guess not.

Pharmacist: Fine, then give us a call when you need a refill. The doctor has authorized six refills for your prescription.

Patient: *(walks away thing to herself)* I have to go through this six more times? I would rather take nothing and take my chances with the diabetes!

Discussion

This pharmacist certainly covered all the necessary information, but the effort was probably counter-productive. Rather than helping the patient get the most benefit from her medication, the pharmacist may have increased the patient's concerns about her condition and medication use, and may actually have discouraged her from taking the medication. If she had considered how the patient was likely to be feeling about a serious and chronic condition like diabetes and about potential problems with medication use, and if she had taken notice of her nonverbal behavior, she may have been more effective in counseling.

Alternate Counseling Situation

Pharmacist: Hello, Mrs. Miller. How are you today?

Patient: *(in a subdued voice)* Oh, I'm OK, I guess.

Pharmacist: *(noticing the patient is subdued and distracted)* You sound a little down today.

Patient: *(sounding worried)* Well yes, I guess I am. The doctors told me that the diet I was on for my sugar wasn't working, and so I have to take pills now.

Pharmacist: *(empathetic tone)* It sounds like you're worried because you're unsure about the need for switching to the pills.

Patient: Yes, I guess it means I'm really a diabetic now, and I know that's really bad. I had a friend whose son had all kinds of problems with it.

Pharmacist: I can see why that would be a worry for you, thinking you might end up with complications like your friend's son. Perhaps it would help if I explained a little about diabetes. *(proceeds to explain about adult-onset diabetes, the potential complications, and the need to keep tight control of blood sugar levels)*

Patient: I see. The doctor did say something about adult diabetes, but I didn't understand. I guess my diabetes must be getting worse if I need this pill now.

Pharmacist: I realize it must seem that way, with the doctor adding the prescription to your diet. Actually, this is a good way of getting better control of your blood sugar than diet alone. I'd like to spend a few minutes now to discuss your prescription to make sure you get the most benefit from it.

Patient: *(sounding interested)* OK. That might help.

Pharmacist: This medication is called glyburide. What did the doctor tell you about it?

Patient: That I should take one every day, and be careful to notice if my blood sugar gets too low. First, I have to worry about it being too high, and now I have to worry about it being too low. How am I supposed to know?

Pharmacist: I realize it sounds like a lot to keep track of. Here's an information sheet that has it all written down. You can read it over at home, then keep it for reference if you forget.

Patient: OK, I'll do that.

Pharmacist: There's some other important things you should know about. Along with the effects on your sugar, glyburide may cause some unwanted effects. These are quite rare, but I want you to be able to recognize them so you can call me right away if you notice anything like this. This information sheet lists the things to look out for. *(points to section of information sheet)*

Patient: OK. As long as I know what to look for, I won't worry so much.

Pharmacist: That's right. Now, did the doctor mention anything about testing your blood regularly for sugar?

Patient: Yes, and she told me to buy a machine to test it.

Pharmacist: Good, because it's an important part of keeping your condidtion under control. *(proceeds to discuss blood glucose monitoring and makes an appointment to teach the patient about using a glucose meter)* I've covered a lot of information fairly quickly. Do you have any questions?

Patient: No, not right now. I'll read this information when I get home.

Pharmacist: Good. I'll be seeing you in a few days to discuss the glucose meter, and we can discuss this information some more then. You have a refill on this prescription to continue on, so I'll be seeing you again in 30 days. We can discuss this further then.

Patient: Thanks so much. *(thinks to herself)* I guess things aren't quite as bad as I thought, after all. I just have to take these pills regularly and test my blood.

Discussion

This time, the pharmacist identified the patient's feelings, understanding that diabetes can be very worrisome to patients. Although there was a lot of information to provide about the medication, the pharmacist acknowledged the patient's feelings and concerns before preceeding. The pharmacist realized that the patient would not be very receptive to information in her worried state of mind.

This identification and response to the patient's feelings was the demonstration of empathy by the pharmacist. By observing the patient's nonverbal language, by listening to the patient, and by identifying her feelings and the meanings of her words, the pharmacist was able to encourage her to discuss her concerns. This in turn gave the pharmacist the opportunity to identify problems and to overcome them. Arranging for follow-up counseling further showed the patient that the pharmacist was genuinely concerned for her welfare. This would encourage further discussion by the patient in future counseling sessions.

Attending to Nonverbal Communication

Nonverbal communication involves all aspects of communication other than spoken or written words, including facial expressions, eye contact, body position, touching, and voice characteristics.[8,15,21,22] In fact, it has been suggested that the impact of any message is comprised of 7% verbal, 38% vocal, and 55% facial communication.[23]

In the situation described earlier, the pharmacist had a surprised look on his face when he heard the patient banging on the counter. Then the pharmacist knocked over the antibiotic and leaned on the counter shaking his head. What did this tell us about the pharmacist? What would it indicate to the patient about the pharmacist's readiness to be empathetic?

Pharmacists' nonverbal language can indicate to patients whether or not they are willing to listen and be empathetic. Nonverbal messages are generally trusted more than verbal, since it is very difficult to lie nonverbally.[22] Thus, even if a pharmacist verbally expresses willingness to help the patient, lack of interest (flat tone of voice, bored facial expression) or haste (quick speech, hurried gestures, frequent glancing away) may be perceived by the patient.

To truly demonstrate concern and willingness to help, the pharmacist must observe a variety of nonverbal cues, including facial expressions, eye contact, body movements and position, voice characteristics and appearance.[8,15,22,23] Appropriate nonverbal behavior for effective patient counseling is illustrated in Table 7.2.

Table 7.2 Nonverbal Behavior for Effective Patient Counseling

Smiling and Friendly Facial Expression: Pharmacist should try to think "pleasant" thoughts before greeting patients because facial expressions reveal feelings.

Varied Eye Contact: Direct contact 50% to 75% of the time to create trust without the discomfort of continual eye contact.

Open and Warm Body Gestures: Raised shoulders and erect head to imply pride and self-esteem, leaning forward to suggest warmth and trust, touching where appropriate to express deep feelings.

Appropriate Distance: 1 1/2 to 4 feet for personal discussion, 4 to 12 feet for impersonal business, avoiding violation of patient's personal space.

Level Position Free of Barriers: Sit or stand beside patient with head at same level, avoiding barriers such as desk or counter.

Moderate and Varied Voice: Rate, pitch, volume appropriate to words and varied to keep interest; indicating "permission" for patient to speak through higher or lower pitch at end of a comment or by silence.

Professional and Clean Appearance: Pharmacist and pharmacy should be neat and clean, pharmacy layout should allow access to pharmacist and privacy.

Adapted from Gerrard BA, Boniface W, Love B. Developing Facilitation Skills. In: Interpersonal Skills for Health Professionals. Reston, VA. 1980. Reston Publishing; Samuelson K. Nonverbal messages can speak louder than words. Health Care. Apr 1986:12-13; Knapp M. Nonverbal Communication: Basic Perspectives, The Effects of Territory and Personal Space. Chapters 1 and 4. In: Essentials of Nonverbal Communication. 2nd ed. New York, 1980. Holt, Rhinehart & Winston.

These nonverbal actions will not be convincing, however, if they are part of an act. Only a genuine feeling of interest and concern for the patient will translate into an effective nonverbal message.

In addition to attending to their own nonverbal communication, pharmacists should observe the patient's nonverbal language.[13] This will assist the pharmacist in identifying the patient's feelings as well as improve patient satisfaction, because studies have found that patients tend to be more satisfied with health-care providers who are skilled at translating nonverbal language to emotional states.[24]

In addition, observation of the patient's nonverbal communication may indicate special needs. For example, a patient with difficulty hearing may turn his head so that his ear is closer, stand closer than normal, or put his hand to his ear. Eyeglasses and hearing aids are also nonverbal indicators that a patient may have special communication needs.

Being Assertive

Another important condition for effective communication in pharmacy practice is the pharmacist's assertiveness. Pharmacists who find it difficult to participate in patient counseling often feel a certain awkwardness in initiating involvement with their patients. Although they will answer patients' questions, they are reluctant to take the first step in communicating. Such pharmacists tend to take comfort in the physical barrier of the pharmacy counter and often allow auxiliary staff to deal with patients. This essentially describes the passive pharmacist.

Conversely, pharmacists who are anxious to get involved in patient counseling sometimes become too aggressive. They insist on counseling each patient regardless of the situation, and tend to force their beliefs and values about medication use and illness on the patient. This kind of behavior inhibits the pharmacist's effectiveness in counseling. As illustration of this, a study of pharmacists during nonprescription counseling observed that pharmacists who were extroverted and aggressive were less likely to persuade the patient to use the product they recommended.[10]

As further illustration of the pitfalls of pharmacists' lack of assertiveness, consider the following patient-counseling scenario.

Counseling Situation

Bill Gregson is a young man who is a regular patient at this pharmacy. Today he is receiving a new prescription for doxycycline 100-mg capsules.

<u>Pharmacist</u>: Hi, Bill! Your prescription is ready. How are you today?

<u>Patient</u>: *(clipped tone)* Fine. How much is it?

<u>Pharmacist</u>: *(ignoring his hurried tone)* I'll just spend a few minutes to go over it with you.

<u>Patient</u>: *(looking irritated)* I'm in a real hurry.

<u>Pharmacist</u>: It'll just take a few minutes. This is an antibiotic, doxycycline...

<u>Patient</u>: *(cuts in, sounding more annoyed now)* Look, the doctor told me all this, and I really have to go. How much is it?

<u>Pharmacist</u>: *(persisting in an authorative tone)* Did he tell you about taking it with food?

<u>Patient</u>: *(sounding frustrated and angry)* No, but I really must go. I've got a job interview across town in 15 minutes. I have to leave right now. Just take my money or give me my prescription back and I'll go elsewhere!

<u>Pharmacist</u>: *(feeling frustrated)* OK. The cashier will take care of you now. Goodbye.

Discussion

The pharmacist began by being aggressive with patient counseling, and thereby aggravated the patient; then the pharmacist became passive, giving up on any attempt to provide important information. The pharmacist was right to attempt to counsel the patient, since it is his responsibility to provide pharmaceutical care. However, an aggressive approach to patient counseling is unlikely to be successful, because counseling requires the patient's cooperation and consent to enter into a two-way discussion. Even if he had managed to give all the necessary information, the patient would not have benefited, since proper discussion to identify and resolve medication-related problems would have been inhibited by the patient's preoccupation, as well as his increasing feelings of frustration and anger.

The passive approach to patient counseling, which the pharmacist finally opted for, was equally ineffective. The patient left without important information and the pharmacist was unable to attempt to discuss real or potential problems with the patient.

The most effective way for the pharmacist to become involved with patients falls somewhere between these two extremes of passivity and aggression. It is an approach known as assertiveness.

Assertiveness "involves standing up for legitimate rights without violating the rights of others or having bad feelings in the process."[25] This allows the pharmacist to express his or her ideas and advice about medication use to patients and other health professionals without infringing on their rights to believe and do what they wish. The result of such an approach is a win–win situation, in which the pharmacist and the other person feel respected and a trusting and mutually respectful relationship can develop.

Reasons for Pharmacists' Nonassertive Behavior

Although the win–win situation resulting from assertiveness is desirable for all, many pharmacists find it difficult to behave assertively.[25] One reason a pharmacist may avoid patient counseling is fear of the patient's rejection of his or her assistance or the patient's anger at being given advice. The assertive pharmacist realizes that although some patients may be unprepared for, or in some way angered by, receiving assistance, he or she can overcome the problem by approaching these patients with empathy and concern, and by explaining the purpose of counseling.

Another concern of the passive pharmacist is that it is a sign of respect to avoid interfering in the patient's affairs. The aggressive pharmacist, on the other hand, believes he is doing patients a favor by "telling" them what to do and feels that everything about a patient is his business. The assertive pharmacist, however, recognizes that although he must consider the patient's point of view and be sensitive to his or her need for privacy, he has a responsibility to "help" the patient get the most benefit from the medication.

Pharmacists may also lack assertiveness as a result of fear of imperfection in themselves.[25] Perfectionist standards can cause them to avoid patient counseling—because it can't always be carried out perfectly. But assertive pharmacists realize that they have a responsibility to help patients, even though they may not always be able to do it exactly as they would wish. Patient counseling and effective communication take practice and are rarely "perfect." Although various circumstances can interfere, and the pharmacist must do everything possible within limitations.

Nonassertive individuals often continue to be passive or aggressive in the belief that their behavior is rooted in an inherent trait. However, individuals can learn to be less passive or less aggressive in their dealings with others through assertiveness training. Assertive behavior will not only improve pharmacists' interactions with patients, but also with employees or employers, co-workers, and other health professionals.

Assertiveness Techniques

The essence of assertive communication is to solve problems in a way that allows both parties to "win." Its aim is not to manipulate people or situations, but to encourage the honest and direct expression of what each party feels and wants. This involves a number of techniques[25]:

1. *Confrontation*: This skill involves letting another person know that he or she is being aggressive, that it is hurting you, and that you will not tolerate it. This can involve simply stating how you *feel* about another's behavior and the *results* of that behavior. For example: "*When you* arrive late for your shift, *I feel* angry *because* then I'm late picking up my son."

   This can be expanded by a specific request of what you want to happen to resolve the situation, "*I'd appreciate it if in future you could* call if you can't make it on time. *This would allow* me to make other arrangements."

   This can be softened by the use of an empathetic statement to start, for example, "I realize that you find it difficult to get here on time."

2. *Saying No:* When another person's request is unreasonable or not possible, the assertive response is to politely refuse. This can be softened by offering an alternative solution. For example, a patient demanding his prescription might be told, "Your doctor is not available to authorize the repeat right now. If your pain is severe, perhaps you could get some treatment in the hospital emergency department."

3. *Making Requests*: When things aren't to your liking, rather than suffering silently, or blowing up and making demands, you are more likely to create a win–win situation if you simply ask someone for what you want.

4. *Expressing Opinions:* Sharing your beliefs and ideas with others can prevent missing out on being involved in a decision or activity. It does not mean that your opinion is forced on others. Opinions should not be forced on others and should preferably include the mention of alternative views.

5. *Initiating Conversations:* Conversation can be initiated with a warm and tactful introduction rather than an abrupt beginning, for example, "Hi, I'm the pharmacist, Susan. I see you're looking at the cough medicines. Can I help you to select one?"

6. *Self-Disclosing*: Although pharmacists expect their patients to give them personal information, they often neglect to act similarly. Building a relationship with a patient can be enhanced by disclosing personal feelings where appropriate (e.g., "I'm sorry your prescription isn't ready. I'm a little slower today because I'm feeling a little under the weather.") This is not to say that excuses should be made regularly, but pharmacists can let patients know that they are people too.

If the pharmacist in the counseling situation discussed earlier had used these assertiveness techniques, he might have been more effective in counseling.

Alternate Counseling Situation

<u>Pharmacist</u>: Hi, Bill! Your prescription is ready. How are you today?

<u>Patient</u>: *(clipped tone)* Fine. How much is it?

<u>Pharmacist</u>: *(recognizing hurried tone)* It's $19.98. The cashier will look after that for you. It sounds like you're in a real hurry.

<u>Patient</u>: *(looking agitated)* Yes, I am.

<u>Pharmacist</u>: *(empathetic tone)* I realize you probably have something important to rush off to, but perhaps you could spare just a few minutes. I need to discuss your prescription with you, to make sure you get the most benefit from it.

<u>Patient</u>: *(sounding calmer, but still hurried)* There's no need. The doctor discussed all that. I've got to get going because I have a job interview across town in 15 minutes.

<u>Pharmacist</u>: *(persisting in an assertive tone)* That sounds really important. What I have to disuss with you is important too, but it can wait until later, perhaps this evening. I'll just give you some printed information for you to read before you take the medication. *(hands over a printed information sheet, pointing to a particular section)* You'll notice that it explains that this medication must be taken with food, or it can upset your stomach. You might want to wait until supper to start.

<u>Patient</u>: *(sounding interested)* Oh, I didn't realize that. I can't afford to have an upset stomach right now.

<u>Pharmacist</u>: I don't want to hold you up any further, but there's more we need to discuss. How about if I call you this evening to go over the information with you?

<u>Patient</u>: That would be fine. Call around seven.

<u>Pharmacist</u>: Fine, I'll do that and good luck with the interview!

<u>Patient</u>: *(rushing off)* Thanks. I'll talk to you tonight.

Discussion

This pharmacist acknowledged the patient's questions about the price right away, allowing the patient to focus his attention on the medication for a minute rather than on paying for the medication. When he responded empathetically to the patient's hurried tone, the patient was encouraged to explain why he was in such a hurry, allowing the pharmacist to recognize immediately that his need to get to the job interview would have to take precedence over counseling. He used the technique of confrontation to explain what he wanted to happen, and he stressed the importance of counseling as a benefit to the patient, not as something that he needed to do for himself. The pharmacist compromised by providing written information and made a specific request of the patient to arrange to continue counseling by telephone later. Although this took about the same amount of time as the previous situation, it resulted in a win–win situation, and both the patient's and the pharmacist's needs were met.

Arranging for Privacy

Privacy is an important condition for effective communication in pharmacy. Patients will not feel comfortable discussing personal topics such as their illnesses in places that they feel others can observe or overhear.[13] Although complete privacy is not necessary, *psychologic* privacy is necessary in which patients can feel that they have the full attention of the pharmacist, and that other patients or pharmacy staff will not be listening.[13] Ways to achieve this will be discussed in Chapter 9.

Displaying a Degree of Emotional Objectivity

When attempting to identify the patient's feelings and the meaning of the patient's words, the pharmacist's own biases and distortions may hinder accurate perception.[17] Personal concerns may cause a pharmacist to be less than fully aware of the patient's feelings. The pharmacist may have certain predetermined ideas about the way a patient should feel in a certain situation.

The situation may arouse the pharmacist's own emotions or cause prejudices toward certain characteristics in the patient to surface, interfering with the ability to identify the patient's feelings accurately.

If the pharmacist is aware that such biases may be present, he or she can attempt to compensate for them by making a conscious effort to remain nonjudgmental and impartial.[17]

This is not to say that the pharmacist should be cold and unfeeling.[13] As mentioned above, it is sometimes appropriate and desirable for the pharmacist to disclose his or her feelings to the patient. However, the pharmacist's feelings should not encroach on the patient's ability to express feelings and needs or on the pharmacist's ability to focus on the patient.[13]

Counseling Skills

A number of skills have been identified as important in conducting a patient-counseling session. They are sometimes referred to as interviewing skills.

As discussed in Chapter 5, the counseling encounter starts with an opening phase, during which it is important for the pharmacist to set a climate for communication with the patient. This is done through the conditions for effective communication discussed above, particularly establishing a helping relationship with the patient and displaying empathy.

The second phase of the counseling encounter involves gathering information and identifying problems. Here, the pharmacist needs skills in listening and probing to fully understand the patient's problems and needs. Other interviewing skills such as paraphrasing, summarizing, transition, and repeating help to keep the discussion flowing smoothly and encourage the patient to become involved.

Listening Skills

The need to listen to a patient would seem to be an obvious element of communication. But pharmacists, in their attempt to cover all the necessary information about medication use, often forget to focus their attention fully on the patient and listen to what he or she has to say and the meaning behind the words. Listening skills fall into four categories: passive listening, acknowledgment responses, encouragement, and active listening.[15]

Passive Listening

Passive listening simply involves allowing the patient to express himself or herself without interference.[15] Pharmacists are often too quick to jump into conversation, denying the patient the opportunity to speak or to finish speaking.

Before telling a patient the purpose of his or her medication, for example, the pharmacist should allow the patient a chance to tell what he or she already knows. This will make counseling more efficient, since the pharmacist may not need to provide any further information; it gives the patient the feeling of being in charge of the situation (an important element in compliance); it allows the pharmacist to detect any misunderstandings; and it may indicate to the pharmacist the kind of language the patient feels comfortable using to describe his or her medication and condition.

As discussed earlier, an important part of empathic responding involves identifying the patient's feelings. While listening passively, the pharmacist can observe the patient's nonverbal language and "read between the lines" to detect the feelings and meanings behind the patient's words.

Acknowledgment Responses

When listening passively, the pharmacist should respond at intervals to let the patient know that he is indeed listening. This may involve simply nodding or uttering expressions such as "Uh-huh."[15]

Encouragement

The pharmacist can also use some words or phrases to encourage the patient to say more about a particular topic.[15] Encouraging phrases may be: "Oh yes." "I see." "Go on." "Tell me more."

Active Listening

Active listening, as the term implies, involves more active participation by the pharmacist. The pharmacist not only makes comments that let the patient know that he is listening and understanding, but takes the opportunity to clarify the patient's feelings and concerns, both for himself and for the patient. This active listening is an essential component of empathetic responding.

Active-listening responses often begin with phrases such as: "You seem to feel...;" "It sounds like you ...;" "I get the sense that you...;" "In other words...;" "As I understand it, you seem to be saying..."[19] Such responses must be made in the appropriate tone of concern or interest; if the pharmacist does not genuinely care about the patient's feelings, this will not sound genuine, and the patient will feel patronized.[15,17]

Active listening should generally be preceded and followed by passive listening, allowing the patient to confirm the feelings that have been identified and discuss concerns at greater length.

Nonlistening Responses

Pharmacists' abilities to listen to their patients are often limited because of behaviors that are counter-productive to listening.[13,15,19] Pharmacists often respond to patients' comments with excessive verbalization, tending to lecture patients rather than engaging them in a discussion, cutting off the patients' expressions of feelings. Pharmacists interrupt patients and monopolize the conversation either because they are in a hurry or because some statement by the patient has caused them to react and interject their own comments. Sometimes, pharmacists simply believe that this behavior constitutes patient counseling and do not realize that the patient may have something to contribute.

Although part of the counseling process involves asking questions, it is inappropriate to ask questions prematurely, before the patient has had an opportunity to express his or her feelings. This tends to remove the focus from the patient and may cause him or her to become defensive. Appropriate questioning should be interspersed with discussion from the patient. This will be discussed in the following section.

Pharmacists sometimes inappropriately evaluate the patient, passing judgment on the situation and the individual involved. This does not help patients; it serves only to discount their feelings and may even make them feel guilty or foolish for having had such feelings or concerns.

A pharmacist's first instinct is often to give advice, since this is an opportunity to show his or her expertise. However, advice is most effective if it is offered after the patient has had an opportunity to finish speaking and explaining his or her problem. And although giving advice is intended to help, it may not be the recommended course of action. In many cases, it is preferable for the pharmacist to encourage patients to explore various avenues themselves, and then to assist them in making decisions.

In an effort to make the patient feel better, and perhaps to make himself or herself feel comfortable, the pharmacist often ignores the feelings expressed by the patient. The pharmacist may do this by changing the subject or by shifting the focus of the discussion from the patient to someone else—often the pharmacist himself or herself or other patients in general. Pharmacists may believe that it will encourage the patient to know that others share their problems. In reality, however, shifting the focus from the patient tends to discount the patient's feelings and may make him or her feel guilty or foolish for having had such concerns.

Although an important part of patient counseling may involve reassuring the patient that the treatment is appropriate and safe, this is inappropriate if it is overly optimistic. Sometimes the pharmacist has no way of being sure if indeed everything will be alright.

Sometimes pharmacists become angry or aggravated with patients' behaviors and respond with hostile comments, sometimes making threatening statements about patients' conditions. Although this understandably happens occasionally, the pharmacist must try to control such feelings. Ways to deal with conflict will be discussed in Chapter 8.

A summary and examples of these nonlistening responses and the appropriate active listening response are shown in Table 7.3. Pharmacists often find it difficult to formulate an active listening response, rather than these nonlistening responses. This takes practice and thought, but can offer the reward of more effective patient counseling.

Probing Skills

After having listened to the patient, the pharmacist may need to probe in order to clarify the problem and determine how he or she can help. Also, during the information-gathering phase of the medication-history interview, the pharmacist needs to probe and ask specific questions about the patient's condition and history.

The way in which these questions are asked is important because it can build, maintain, or destroy rapport between the pharmacist and the patient.[20,26] To be effective, questions asked by the pharmacist must obtain accurate information, obtain the information efficiently, and involve the patient as much as possible.[20,26]

The skills used in asking effective questions during counseling involve the organization and phrasing of questions. This is the essence of probing skills.[20,26]

Table 7.3 Nonlistening Responses

In response to the patient's statement, "The dentist told me I'd have to come back again next week. I just wonder if he knows what he's doing." *the pharmacist may make one of the following responses:*

Excessive Verbalization: "Well, the prescription the dentist gave you looks fine. It's for an analgesic to help the pain. Take it every 4 hours...etc."

Premature Questioning: "What were your symptoms when you saw the dentist? Did he take any X-rays?"

Being Evaluative: "You're just feeling bad because of the pain. If you had regular check-ups you wouldn't be in such a bad state now."

Advising: "You should see another dentist if you feel that way."

Ignoring the Patient's Feelings: "Lots of people have problems with their teeth and have to return to their dentists for treatment. I had an abscessed tooth, and it took weeks to clear up."

Reassuring: "I'm sure the dentist knows what he's doing, and everything will be just fine."

Hostile: "Well, that's just plain unfair to the dentist. Anyway, you'd better do what he says or you'll end up losing that tooth."

An Active Listening Response would be: "I guess you're pretty frustrated at having to go back to the dentist again."

Adapted from Gerrard BA, Boniface W, Love B. Developing Facilitation Skills. In: Interpersonal Skills for Health Professionals. Reston, VA: Reston Publishing, 1980:133-136.

Organization of Questions

Questioning should be introduced with a statement regarding the purpose in order to prevent the patient from becoming defensive. For example, to introduce questioning during nonprescription counseling the pharmacist may say, "I need to ask you some questions about your symptoms to determine which medication would be most effective for you."

Because patients may feel more comfortable later in the interview once more trust has been developed, the pharmacist should begin with less personal questions and proceed to more personal questions, such as details of the patient's alcohol use.

To explore where the questioning should focus, the pharmacist should start with more general questions and become more specific as the direction becomes clear, for example, "What sort of cold symptoms do you have?"... "Is there also a cough?"... "Is the cough dry?"

Finally, questions should be grouped together by topic to allow both the pharmacist and the patient to focus attention on a particular area, likely resulting in better patient recall. For example, during a medication-history interview, the pharmacist should ask all relevant questions about a particular drug before proceeding to questions about the next drug.

Phrasing of Questions

The way that questions are phrased may also contribute to their effectiveness.[20,26]

Open questions, which demand more than a "yes" or "no" answer, encourage the patient to explain his or her point of view, and to express problems in his own terms. They are formulated using words such as how, when, where, what, or who.

Open questions are particularly useful at the beginning of the interview to elicit as much information from the patient as possible. They can also assist information gathering by encouraging more discussion by the patient, such as "Tell me more about that?"

Closed questions are those that require only a "yes" or "no" response and tend to elicit mostly factual information. They are useful for gathering specific information about a particular problem and fill in the gaps left by the open-ended questions. For example, if the patient has reported that the medication seems to cause an upset stomach, the pharmacist might ask, "Do you take this medication with food?" The judicious use of a variety of open and closed questions will result in the most effective gathering of information.

Questions that begin with "why" should be avoided, because they may elicit defensiveness and are less likely to gather accurate information. "Why" questions tend to elicit what the patient believes to be a socially acceptable answer rather than the truth either because they don't want to reveal the truth or they aren't sure of the answer. For example, when questioning a patient about noncompliance, rather than asking, "Why aren't you taking this medication?", the pharmacist should first ask, "How are you taking this medication?"and then, "What problems are you having taking this medication?"

Certain phrasing of questions may lead to bias in the patient's answers. Leading questions that suggest the expected answer or restrictive questions that dissuade the patient from providing a truthful response should be avoided. Rather than asking, "You do take this medication the way your doctor told you to, don't you?", the pharmacist should ask, "How are you taking this medication?"

Two-sided questions that solicit more than one item of information should be avoided, since this will lead to confusion. The patient will not know which part to answer first, and the pharmacist may not know which question is being answered. In addition, the other questions will probably have to be repeated or will be forgotten.

Finally, questions should be tactful and never unnecessarily personal or prying. The pharmacist should ask only necessary questions and consider the patient's personal situation (e.g., marital or employment status) so as to avoid embarrassing the patient or putting him or her on the defensive.

A summary of these probing skills is presented in Table 7.4.

Table 7.4   Probing Skills

Organization of Questions

Introduce questions

Proceed from less to more personal

Proceed from general to specific

Group questions together by topic

Phrasing of Questions

Appropriate use of open and closed questions

Minimizing "Why" questions

Avoid questions that lead to bias

Avoid double-barrelled questions

Questions should be tactful and should avoid unnecessary prying

Adapted from Gardner M, Boyce R, Herrier R. Pharmacist-Patient Consultation Program. 1991. U.S.A., U.S. Public Health Service, Indian Health Service; Bernstein L, Bernstein RS. The Probing Response. In: Interviewing: A Guide for Health Professionals. 4th ed. 1985. New York, Appleton-Century Crofts.

Other Interviewing Skills

A number of other interviewing skills can help the pharmacist to be efficient and effective in counseling. Paraphrasing is a helpful technique for the pharmacist to verify his or her understanding of the patient.[20] Intermittently, as necessary, the pharmacist might simply re-state what he or she believes the patient has said. As well as verifying the facts, re-stating answers or paraphrasing lets the patient know that the pharmacist has been paying attention. For example, in response to the patient's statement, "This pain in my kidneys is so bad I can hardly stand up." The pharmacist might respond, "Are you saying the pain in your lower back makes it difficult for you to straighten?" Paraphrasing is also part of empathetic responding, which was discussed earlier, and can help to calm and focus the patient's thoughts.

Summarizing is a useful technique to end a series of probing questions.[20] This helps the pharmacist to clarify what problems have been identified before going on to discuss those problems. For example, "It seems from what you've told me that you find the medication is helping with your arthritis pain, but that it upsets your stomach a little." If this summary is incorrect, the patient can then inform the pharmacist and provide additional information if necessary.

Repeating the patient's words in the form of questions is another technique that encourages the patient to talk more about a particular topic.[14] For example, in response to the patient's comments about pain in the kidney, the pharmacist might say, "A pain in your kidneys?" This should not be done too frequently or it could become annoying.

Sometimes the pharmacist needs to use a transition statement to switch the discussion to a different topic, for example, from discussion of the patient's conditions to the medications used.[14] This is also useful when the patient intervenes with comments on another topic. After discussing that briefly, the pharmacist needs to return to the topic at hand. For example, the pharmacist might say, "Your holiday sounds like it was terrific, but now I'd like to talk about how you managed to take your heart pills while you were away."

Communicating with Peers

During the course of their daily activities, pharmacists communicate not only with patients but also with other pharmacy personnel such as pharmacists, pharmacy technicians, clerks, delivery people, sales representatives, order-desk clerks, etc. Pharmacists also communicate daily with other health professionals such as physicians, dentists, nurses, and various community health workers (home-visiting nurses, public-health nurses, social workers, and home-care workers). In order to provide optimal pharmaceutical care as well as to find the time to counsel patients, pharmacists need to communicate well with all of these people.

Interactions with other health professionals and pharmacy personnel are often hurried, and occasionally are confrontational. These relationships are affected by a variety of stresses. Pharmacists will therefore find it useful to explore the nature of these interactions and develop more effective ways of dealing with their co-workers and colleagues in the health-care team.

Difficulties Dealing with Peers

Pharmaceutical care requires pharmacists to be involved in identifying and resolving medication-related problems and to be jointly responsible for the outcomes of therapy.[27] This means that pharmacists will need to be involved more than ever in discussion with other health professionals, particularly physicians, sometimes under difficult circumstances, (e.g., when a patient outcome has been negative or when the pharmacist has detected a problem involving the physician's prescribing).

A recent survey of pharmacists found that physicians were cooperative 96% of the time when pharmacists contacted them to recommend another product or strength, ask for clarification, or correct an error.[28] However, pharmacists do sometimes find physician–pharmacist relations to be strained, and may find this increasingly so as they become more involved in the patient's therapy and treatment outcomes. Hepler and Strand have pointed out that pharmaceutical care must be integrated with the other elements of care in order to benefit the patient fully, but that cooperation is complicated by the possibility that pharmaceutical care represents an expansion into the traditional roles of physicians and nurses.[27]

The main sources of pharmacists' difficulties dealing with other health professionals have been found to include struggles for power, poor communication, and an unsatisfactory communication environment.[1] These difficulties can equally apply to problems between pharmacists and other pharmacy personnel.

Struggles for power and autonomy have been identified as the main barriers to communication between pharmacists and other health professionals.[1] In a survey of pharmacist–physician relationships, physicians "applauded" pharmacists' competence and professionalism and their "watchdog" services over drug use, but they disliked pharmacists' recommending products and saw this as an encroachment on their "turf."[27]

Another source of pharmacists' problems in dealing with other health professionals has been identified as poor communication between professionals.[1] Studies suggest that pharmacists are aware of this problem.[30,31] Part of the communication problem may simply be that too little communication occurs. In survey responses, physicians do not generally identify community pharmacists as sources of information about medications, although they consider hospital pharmacists to be their primary source for such information.[29] The nature of the communication that does occur constitutes another aspect of the problem. Other health professionals have different issues, priorities, and concerns that may differ from those of pharmacists or so they believe.[30] Physicians sometimes perceive that pharmacists are only concerned with reducing costs rather than optimal patient care.[30] Greater exposure to services by pharmacists tends, however, to improve physicians' attitudes toward pharmacists.[31]

The environment in which pharmacists generally have to deal with other health professionals may be another source of difficulties.[1] The hospital and community pharmacy environment often lacks privacy, so that any altercations or reprimands can be overheard by others, adding to the degree of discomfort for the individual involved. There is often interference and background noise, even during telephone conversations, as well as many distractions and the pressure of time.

Interaction between pharmacists and their peers often occurs over the telephone, and this medium tends to accentuate the distance between the parties involved. Telephone communication has been identified by both physicians and pharmacists as a source of aggravation.[29] Physicians dislike waiting on the telephone or getting busy signals, and pharmacists are irritated by having to deal with receptionists and having to make unnecessary phone calls to physicians.[29]

Much of the communication between physicians and pharmacists occurs in the writing of prescriptions. Surprisingly, physicians seem to be more sensitive about this problem than pharmacists: 50% (compared with only 10% of pharmacists) report that their illegible handwriting is one source of the problems they experience with pharmacists.[29] Written forms and notes are also used between pharmacy personnel and between pharmacists and other health professionals. These forms can sometimes be perceived negatively, because they are impersonal and often poorly worded so that recommendations are perceived as demands, or reports of problems are perceived as blame.

Improving Pharmacist–Peer Relations

Pharmacists can work at improving their relationships with other health professionals and pharmacy personnel by improving the frequency and content of communication, by demonstrating empathy for peers, and by being assertive with peers.

Improving the Content of Communication

The problem of differing issues, concerns, and priorities for different health professionals and pharmacy personnel can be overcome by bringing the focus to the patient.[30,32] Since this should be the concern for all involved, making any suggestion by framing it in terms of how it will benefit patient care will remove the focus from individual health professional's behavior and reduce confrontation and arguments.

Providing a high level of service to other health professionals cannot help but improve relations. Pharmacists can improve their level of service by making sure to do the following:[29,32]

- Being available to answer questions in a timely and dependable manner;
- Taking the time to explain problems with data and references to support the advice rather than informing the health professional that an error has been made;
- Suggesting alternatives rather than one recommendation, allowing the health professional to make an informed decision rather than feeling as if he or she has been dictated to;
- Continuing to provide services such as warnings of potential drug abuse/ misuse, prescription errors, and drug interactions and by keeping patient profiles;
- Monitoring patient treatment and providing feedback to other health professionals involved regarding the patient's progress;
- Providing proper documentation of actions taken with patients to let other health professionals know that pharmacists are indeed performing these functions.

Conflicts between pharmacists and other health professionals often arise when pharmacists make recommendations.[33] Therefore, conflict resolution and negotiation techniques should be used by pharmacists to resolve these types of issues.[33] Some suggestions have been made by Szeinback for avoiding conflict when making recommendations to colleagues including:[45]

- Factual information should be reported in a clear, concise and organized manner;
- The way in which the recommendation decreases risk or improves care for the patient should be explained clearly;
- Flexibility and willingness to admit a lack of understanding should be displayed;
- Criticism of colleagues should be avoided;
- Feedback should be used to make sure that others understand and to encourage questions and comments.

Improving the Frequency of Communication

One way for pharmacists to increase the frequency of communication with other health professionals is for pharmacists to mount an active campaign to promote pharmacy services. Pharmacists should consider meeting regularly with the health professionals with whom they deal. For example, when starting in a new practice, pharmacists should take the initiative to introduce themselves in person (or by telephone as a second choice) to health professionals with whom they will be dealing. New health professionals who move into the area should be contacted. This introduction should include personal information about the pharmacist as well as his or her practice approach, services she or he will provide, and an assurance that his or her concerns, like the health professionals, are based on securing the best possible health care for the patient.

Pharmacists can create forums for communication with other health professionals by organizing seminars on drug information. Orientation programs to pharmacy services can be organized to improve communication between pharmacy personnel and others such as nurses.[34]

Pharmacists can also communicate with peers through written, facsimile, or telephone consultations. Providing a newsletter and written reports of pharmaceutical interventions can let health professionals know that pharmacists are knowledgeable and are performing a valuable service. Careful attention should be made, however, when preparing written communication so that the message is not misinterpreted, as this can be a source of problems as discussed earlier. This will be discussed in the next section on written communication.

Since the environment of the communication can contribute to problems, attention should be given to this. Attempts should be made to have conversations in private, or at least away from the main stream of activities. Regular meetings should be arranged (e.g., staff meetings, pharmacy–nursing meetings, etc.) so that concerns can be aired, and so that positive feedback can be given to the group for co-operative work.

Empathizing with Peers

Pharmacists can improve relations with peers by displaying empathy with health professionals and colleagues in the same way that they do with patients. By letting the other person know that his or her point of view has been understood, the pharmacist can reduce tensions and lead the way to better problem solving together in a more equal partnership.

Consider a nurse telephoning the hospital pharmacist to check on a missing medication. The nurse's first priority is to get the dose to the patient on time. She is probably very rushed, is worried about the patient, and is worried about being held responsible for any problems resulting from a missed dose. If the pharmacist responds to her query by defensively accusing her of not sending down the order or by complaining that he too is busy, conflict is sure to arise. Alternatively, the pharmacist can empathize with the nurse's situation and let her know that her needs will be addressed as soon as possible. He can then proceed to ask any questions that might be necessary to solve the problem, and suggest possible solutions.

Being Assertive with Peers

Assertiveness on the pharmacist's part can also help to develop better peer relationships. Pharmacists who are tentative and unsure of themselves in their communications with peers are not likely to receive respect. Recall that assertiveness involves giving and receiving respect and creating a win–win situation.

By being assertive, the pharmacist can ensure that his or her point of view gains recognition while at the same time letting colleagues know that their view is receiving equal consideration. This too will lead the way to focusing on the patient's problem and solving it together in a rational way, for the patient's benefit. Pharmacists may sometimes need to remind peers that it is the patient who is at issue and on whom the discussion should focus—rather than on either of the colleagues.

Improving Pharmacist–Employee Relations

Because pharmacists are often in a supervisory capacity in the pharmacy, they also need to be aware of communication aspects particular to the employee–employer relationship. Good relationships in this quarter will allow the pharmacist to concentrate on patients' concerns, by freeing up time and mental capacity, as well as reducing stress in the pharmacy environment.

Building and maintaining an effective employee–employer relationship takes time and patience.[35] The communication skills discussed with respect to dealing with patients and with peers apply equally here including empathetic responding, active listening, and assertiveness. Some guidelines to foster good employee–employer relationships have been suggested by Sepinwell:[35]

- Clear rules should be set and consistently enforced;
- Mistakes should be admitted;

- Employees should be involved in planning and encouraged to be creative;
- Power of decision making and conflict resolution should be shared where possible;
- Individuals should not be required to do more than they are able;
- Employees should be shown that they are trusted;
- Problems identified should be a result of an employee's actions, not the individual person;
- The good in what the person is doing should be discussed along with the bad;
- Comparisons between employees and favoritism should be avoided;
- Honest expression of feelings should be encouraged for management and employees;
- Kindness and consideration should be observed.

Telephone and Written Communication

A significant portion of pharmacists' communication with patients and health professionals is conducted over the telephone and in writing. Since this form of communication does not involve face-to-face contact, there is less of a nonverbal component to assist in transmitting the message, allowing a greater opportunity for misinterpretation. Pharmacists should be aware of the potential for problems and attempt to overcome them through various communication techniques.

Telephone Communication

Pharmacists spend a good part of their day on the telephone talking to physicians and patients. Although there are some commonalities, there are specific points to consider when dealing with patients as compared with health professionals.

Telephone Communication with Patients

Although most patient counseling is conducted in person, pharmacists are advised to conduct patient counseling over the telephone for situations where the patient cannot be present in the pharmacy, where the patient or pharmacist are limited by time, or where the situation demands a level of privacy that is not available in the pharmacy. In addition, patients often call the pharmacy to ask questions and place orders.

Sometimes, a telephone call is the patient's first interaction with the pharmacy and a particular pharmacist, and therefore may be important in developing rapport for future interactions.

A number of suggestions have been made for improving telephone communication with patients.[36,37] These and some additional considerations can improve the pharmacist's efficiency and effectiveness in conducting patient counseling by telephone:

1. *Be Prepared.* If the pharmacist is initiating a telephone interview, the pharmacist should be prepared with the patient's drug profile and any additional information they wish to provide. If the patient initiates the phone call, then the patient's name should be ascertained and used during the call and the patient's drug profile should be retrieved so that complete information is available during the discussion.

2. *Deal with Patients Promptly.* There should be a prearranged plan of whom should answer the telephone with an allowance for backup after two to three rings if that person is not available. If the patient must wait for the pharmacist, the clerk answering the telephone should indicate that the pharmacist is with a patient and will come to the phone as soon as possible. If it appears that it will be a lengthy wait, the clerk should indicate this and if possible arrange for the pharmacist to call the patient back. If the patient must be put "on hold," the patient should be told why and asked if they would hold, then should be thanked for waiting when the conversation is resumed.

3. *Start with a Friendly Greeting.* The pharmacist should try to smile when speaking on the telephone to transmit a friendly attitude through his or her voice. Whether the pharmacist or patient initiates the phone call, the pharmacist should greet the patient and identify his or her pharmacy, name and title.

4. *Avoid Interruptions.* The pharmacist should try to ensure that he or she is not interrupted while on the telephone with a patient, and try to remove distraction so that the patient can be given her or his full attention.

5. *Maintain Confidentiality.* The patient's confidentiality should be maintained by ensuring that the telephone conversation cannot be overheard by other pharmacy customers. The pharmacist should also be careful when telephoning the patient that the patient's situation is not discussed with anyone in the household other than the patient.

6. *Follow the Appropriate Counseling Protocol.* As with any patient-counseling session, the interview should follow the appropriate protocol as discussed in Chapter 5.

7. *Compensate for the Decrease in Nonverbal Communication.* Since nonverbal communication is reduced, the pharmacist should be alert for the patient's tone of voice and speech rhythms to detect concerns or lack of understanding. The pharmacist can compensate by using good verbal descriptions and a variety of terms. Also, if a pause is made to write or think, some sound or indication should be made to let the caller know this.

8. *Conclude by Asking if the Patient Has Anything Further to Discuss.* Since the pharmacist cannot see any hesitation on the caller's part, it is particularly important that the interview be concluded by asking if the patient has any questions or anything further to discuss.

9. *Offer to Make a Follow-up Call*. As with the face-to-face counseling protocol, the pharmacist should offer to telephone the caller later for follow-up if necessary to make sure everything was understood.
10. *End on a Positive Note*. To close the telephone call, the pharmacist should try to end on a positive note, particularly if a problem is still unsolved, for example, "I've tried my best to help. Please call again." The pharmacist should not hang up until he or she is sure that the patient is indeed finished speaking.
11. *Document*. Telephone counseling should be documented on the patient's profile in the same way as any patient-counseling interview would be, to note any problems identified and interventions recommended.

Telephone Communication with Health Professionals

As discussed above, telephone conversations can be a source of problems between pharmacists and health professionals. However, if appropriate communication skills are used, telephone communication can be an effective way to increase communication with health professionals.

Some suggestions have been made to make telephone conversations with physicians more efficient.[37] These and some additional suggestions follow:

1. *Arrange for a Private Line*. A separate telephone line should be used only for health professionals, and answered by a pharmacist to ensure quick and direct response to telephone calls from health professionals.
2. *Observe Telephone Manners*. Telephone manners as recommended above should be observed when answering the telephone, putting on hold, and hanging up.
3. *Be Prepared*. The pharmacist should be prepared when telephoning a physician by having appropriate patient information and well-thought-out recommendations, alternatives, and supporting data.
4. *Be Brief but Friendly*. Conversations should be brief and to the point, but should not be curt. After clearly identifying himself (e.g., name, pharmacy), the pharmacist should spend a moment exchanging pleasantries. This should be brief, but should not be omitted, because it can help to build an interpersonal relationship.
5. *State the Purpose of the Call*. The purpose of the call should be stated clearly, to signal that it is time for business. This will also help the health professional prepare mentally, as well as to take the time to retrieve the patient chart or any other material necessary. The purpose should include the patient's name as well as any other identification generally used specific to the practice (e.g., chart number, clinic or office patient, from hospital emergency visit, etc.). If it is anticipated that the purpose of the call might lead to a lengthy discussion, the pharmacist should state this and allow the health professional to arrange an alternate time if necessary.

6. *Show Respect for All Members of the Patient's Health Care Team.* Often the pharmacist has to speak with a nurse or receptionist before being allowed to speak with the physician. These people are part of the health-care team, since they are usually familiar with the patient as well, and therefore, should not be ignored or treated with a lack of respect. Building interpersonal relationships with all involved in the patient's care will ultimately improve the patient's care. Of course, care should be taken regarding confidentiality.

7. *Be Empathetic and Assertive.* Skills of empathy and assertiveness should be remembered when dealing on the telephone. For example, often when a pharmacist telephones a physician's office, the office is very busy, and the physician may even be with a patient when she takes the call. This may make it difficult for her to concentrate on the patient the pharmacist wishes to discuss. By using empathetic skills, the pharmacist can let the health professional know that he recognizes that this may be the case.

   The pharmacist may need to use assertive skills to make sure that the receptionist or nurse will allow the pharmacist to speak with the physician. Assertiveness may also be needed to ensure that the pharmacist's concerns or recommendations are considered by the physician.

8. *Summarize.* The telephone conversation should be summarized with a clear statement of what will be done, if anything.

9. *End on a Positive Note.* The pharmacist should try to end the conversation on a positive note, even if the situation was not resolved. Without being solicitous, the pharmacist should thank the health professional for his or her time.

Written Communication

As discussed in Chapter 6, written information has become a mainstay of providing information to patients, although it should always be used together with verbal discussion, either before or after the patient has read the material. As discussed previously, this material should be prepared and used with consideration for appropriate content, readability and comprehension, and presentation format.

Written communication is used between pharmacy personnel and between pharmacists and other health professionals, and includes notes, forms, and prescriptions. This kind of communication tends to be impersonal and often is poorly worded. As a result, the message is often interpreted negatively, for example, recommendations made in writing are perceived as demands for change, or reports of problems are perceived as accusations.

To avoid communication problems, written communication should be carefully organized and worded to avoid any suggestion that orders are being given, or blame is being placed for errors. Such forms as intervention forms, incident reports, performance reviews, etc. should be planned with input from all who will be using and receiving them. A personal note added, in the form of a greeting and comments in hand writing by the sender, can help to soften the effect of forms and form letters.

Summary

This chapter provided only a brief review of communication aspects of pharmacy practice. Pharmacists should seek more in-depth understanding of these topics through readings and workshops when they are available (see Appendix A). Practice is the most beneficial way to improve communication skills, and pharmacists should try to develop these skills over time.

Although this chapter discussed communication with patients in general, as well as with peers, there are specific kinds of communication difficulties that arise. These will be discussed in the next chapter with respect to tailoring counseling for the individual patient.

References

1. Kimberlin C. Communications. In: Pharmacy Practice: Social and Behavioral Aspects. 3d ed. Wertheimer A, Smith MC, eds. Baltimore, Williams & Wilkins. 1989.
2. Ley P. Techniques for increasing patients' recall and understanding. In: Communicating with Patients: Improving Communication Satisfaction and Compliance. New York: Croom Helm. 1988.
3. Waitzkin H. Doctor-patient communication: Clinical implications of social scientific research. JAMA. 1984;252(17):2441-2446.
4. Davis H, Fallowfield L. Counseling theory. In: Counseling and Communication in Health Care. Davis H, Fallowfield L, eds. Chichester, England: John Wiley & Sons. 1991.
5. Berger B, McCroskey J, Baldwin JH. Cognitive change in pharmacy communication courses: Need and assessment. Am J Pharm Educ. 1986;59(1):51-55.
6. Watkins RL, Norwood GJ, Meister FL. Improving the quality of the pharmacist as a drug advisor to patients and physicians through continuing education. Am J Pharm Educ. 1976;40:34-39.
7. Gerrard BA, Boniface W, Love B. Developing skills in understanding interpersonal behavior. In: Interpersonal Skills for Health Professionals. Reston, VA: Reston Publishing. 1980.
8. Lively B. Communication as a transactional process—Basic tools of the community pharmacist. Contemp Pharm Pract. 1978;1(2):81-85.
9. Lawrence G. People Types and Tiger Stripes: A Practical Guide to Learning Styles. 2nd Ed. Gainsville, Fla: Center for Application of Psychological Type. 1982:13-25.
10. Nichol M, McCombs J, Johnson K, et al. The effects of consultation on over-the-counter medication purchasing decisions. Med Care. 1992;30(11):989-1003.

11. Dusay J, Dusay K, Transactional analysis. In: Current Psychotherapies. 3rd ed. Corsini R and contributors. Itasca, IL: FE Peacock Publishers, Inc. 1984.
12. Elder J. Introduction to the Ego States. In: Transactional Analysis in Health Care. Menlo Park, CA: Addison-Wesley Publishing Co. 1978.
13. Bernstein L, Bernstein RS. An overview of interviewing techniques. In: Interviewing: A Guide for Health Professionals. 4th Ed. New York: Appleton-Century-Crofts. 1985.
14. Reiser DE, Klein A. The interview process. In: Patient Interviewing—The Human Dimension. Baltimore, Waverly Press, 1980.
15. Gerrard BA, Boniface W, Love B. Developing Facilitation Skills. In: Interpersonal Skills for Health Professionals. Reston, VA: Reston Publishing. 1980.
16. Montagne M. Research and evaluation in health communication. Am J Pharm Ed. 1987;51(3):172-177.
17. Barnard D, Barr J, Schumacher G. Empathy. Person to Person. The AACP-Lilly Pharmacy Communications Skills Project. Bethesda, MD: American Association of Colleges of Pharmacy. 1982.
18. Meach B, Rogers C. Person-centred therapy. In: Current Psychotherapies. 3rd ed. Corsini R and Contributors. Itasca, IL: FE Peacock Publishers. 1984.
19. Bernstein L, Bernstein RS. The understanding response. In: Interviewing: A Guide for Health Professionals. 4th Ed. New York: Appleton-Century-Crofts. 1985.
20. Gardner M, Boyce R, Herrier R. Pharmacist-Patient Consultant Program. An Interactive Approach to Verify Patient Understanding. U.S. Public Health Service, Indian Health Service. 1991.
21. Knapp M. Nonverbal Communication: Basic Perspectives. In: Essentials of Nonverbal Communication. New York: Holt, Rhinehart & Winston. 1980.
22. Samuelson K. Non-verbal messages can speak louder than words. Health Care. Apr 1986:12-13.
23. Knapp M. The effects of territory and personal space. In: Essentials of Nonverbal Communication. New York: Holt, Rhinehart & Winston. 1980.
24. DiMatteo MR, Taranta A, Friedman HS, et al. Predicting patient satisfaction from physicians' non-verbal communication skills. Med Care. 1980;18(4):376-387.
25. Gerrard BA, Boniface W, Love B. Developing assertion skills. In: Interpersonal Skills for Health Professionals. Reston, VA: Reston Publishing. 1980.
26. Bernstein L, Bernstein RS. The probing response. In: Interviewing: A Guide for Health Professionals. 4th Ed. New York: Appleton-Century-Crofts. 1985.
27. Hepler C, Strand L. Opportunities and responsibilities in pharmaceutical care. Am J Hosp Pharm. 1990;47(3):533-543.
28. Meade V. APhA survey look at patient counseling. Am Pharm. 1992;NS32(4):27-29.

29. Anon. 1984 Schering Report explores pharmacist-physician relationships. Am Pharm. 1984;24(10):13-14.

30. Albro W. How to communicate with physicians. Am Pharm. 1993;NS33(4):59-61.

31. Ritchey FJ, Raney MR. Effect of exposure on physicians' attitudes toward clinical pharmacists. Am J Hosp Pharm.38:1459-1463.

32. Timmerman S. How to work with physicians. Am Pharm.1992;NS32(2): 39-40.

33. Szeinbach S. Helpful ideas: Using interpersonal skills to resolve conflicts with prescribers.The Cons Pharm.1991;6(6):524,526.

34. Welch P, Wright P, Harell A, et al. Development of a pharmacy/nursing orientation program. Abstract of Meeting Presentation. ASHP Midyear Clinical Meeting. 26 1991: p127D.

35. Sepinwell S. Managing to communicate. The Leading Edge.1992;2(3):8,9.

36. Smith DL. Communicating with patients by telephone. Am Pharm. 1983; NS23(10):38.

37. Hunter R. Effective Telephone communication. In: Communication in Pharmacy Practice. Tindall WN, Beardsley RS, Curtis FR, eds. Philadelphia: Lea & Febiger. 1984.

8
TAILORING COUNSELING

After studying the counseling protocols suggested in Chapter 5, a pharmacist or pharmacy student may respond: "I see the idea behind the protocol for counseling and basic counseling techniques, but will that apply to all situations? What about counseling a disabled person, or an elderly patient?" Although these protocols should generally be followed, the content of the counseling needs to be varied. Certain points in the counseling may need to be emphasized, and the various materials, methods, and techniques used in counseling may need to be altered. Tailoring the counseling protocol in this way can assist the pharmacist in dealing with a variety of difficulties while being efficient and effective in counseling.

Factors to Be Considered in Tailoring Counseling

Pharmacists have reported that many factors contribute to difficulties in patient counseling.[1] These factors include characteristics of the patient, the type of drug or condition being treated, and various aspects of the situation.

Characteristics of the Patient

Certain patient characteristics will affect the emphasis that needs to be placed on certain aspects of counseling. The age of the patient may affect counseling in a number of ways. Elderly patients may use multiple drugs to treat several conditions and may experience unexpected reactions to medications resulting from the physiological changes of aging.[2] The pharmacist may therefore have to spend more time than he or she would with another patient identifying problems, explaining directions, and helping the patient schedule dosing.[2] Similarly, pediatric patients require more attention regarding problem identification because of their physiological differences from adults. More time will also likely be required for providing detailed instructions to the caregiver about administration.[3]

The cultural background of the patient may also alter the emphasis in counseling. People with different cultural backgrounds may have different perceptions of their illnesses and of the purpose or effectiveness of medication.[4] For example, some Europeans are more accustomed to using herbal remedies, and they may have doubts about the effectiveness of prescribed medications.

The type of information provided in terms of detail and selection of patient education materials may also need to be varied depending on the patient's abilities and preferences as discussed in Chapter 6.

Some patients may also have various disabilities that may affect where counseling can take place, the patient-education materials used, and the type of information that may be needed.[5]

A patient's type of employment and lifestyle may need to be considered. The dosage form, dosing schedule, and side effects may need to be modified, and special arrangements may need to be made. For example, a truck driver will have difficulty taking a medication that makes him drowsy.

The patient's gender, employment status, or socio-economic situation should *not* alter the type of counseling provided; however, these factors should be considered by the pharmacist during certain discussions in order to prevent embarrassing or offending the patient.

Characteristics of the Drug

As discussed earlier, the content of the counseling will vary depending on whether a prescription or a nonprescription drug is involved. Also, certain drugs are more likely than others to present problems with compliance, side effects, or precautions.

Where a drug is known to be associated with a high risk of interactions or adverse effects, this section in the protocol should be emphasized. Other medications, such as those administered by inhalation or injection, may require more emphasis on the method of use.

Another consideration with regard to the drug may be the length of time that it will take before a patient will recognize an effect, as with some antidepressants, or the lack of evident effect, as with antihypertensives. As discussed in Chapter 4, it is important in these situations to help the patient find ways to identify the medication effect in some way (e.g., through suggesting self-monitoring of blood pressure) to encourage compliance.

Characteristics of the Condition

Some conditions may arouse more confusion or concern for the patient than others.[4] For example, the diagnosis and prognosis of high blood pressure are often poorly understood. Similarly, a diagnosis of epilepsy may cause a patient embarrassment and worry about other people's reactions. In particular, where the illness may be terminal, such as cancer or AIDS, the patient will have a variety of concerns and emotions requiring special attention by the pharmacist.

The pharmacist may need to spend more time in such cases discussing the condition with the patient, and the patient's feelings. When counseling patients with these conditions, it is also important to emphasize how the medication works in relation to controlling or reducing symptoms rather than curing the condition, and the consequences of missing a dose of the medication without, of course, resorting to scare tactics.

Characteristics of the Situation

Different situations will also call for different emphasis in counseling. As discussed in Chapter 5, the content of the counseling will vary, depending on whether the patient is new to the pharmacy or is a returning patient.

A situation in which a patient becomes angry, fearful, or emotionally upset can make counseling particularly difficult for the pharmacist. The pharmacist will need to deal with the patient's emotions before the counseling can proceed.

Difficult situations also arise when the patient's aims are in conflict with the pharmacist's, for example, when the patient is particularly in a hurry, or alternatively, wanting to talk more with the pharmacist than necessary.

Pharmacists are also presented with difficulties as a result of the pharmacy environment. In particular, interruptions during counseling can pose problems. There are many other barriers for pharmacists regarding patient counseling, and these will be discussed further in Chapter 9.

Finally, pharmacists are often consulted by patients with a range of social concerns from child abuse to threatened suicide. Although these situations do not require medication counseling, the pharmacist is required, because of his or her position in the community, to respond to such situations.

Tailoring Counseling to Overcome Difficulties

Counseling must be tailored to accommodate factors that have the potential to impede the progress of counseling. Pharmacists may make appointments with certain groups of patients with special needs, therefore requiring more detailed counseling.[6] Pharmacists may choose to start with patients they believe to be at greatest risk of medication-related problems, or patient groups who are most prevalent in the community.

It should be recognized at the outset of this discussion, that the patients in these difficult situations in *no way* form homogeneous groups, and that each patient should be considered on an individual basis. In addition, it must be emphasized that *the patient himself is not a problem*, just his circumstances in relation to the pharmacist's concerns regarding patient counseling.

Counseling Patients with Poor Language Comprehension

As discussed in Chapter 6, pharmacists are often confronted with language barriers of various sorts when counseling patients. These can include not only the obvious barrier of a foreign language, but also the more subtle barriers to comprehension due to the pharmacist's use of jargon and technical phrases, or the patient's low literacy level.

Sometimes pharmacists are not aware of the problem, because people with language difficulties are often skilled at concealing their difficulties.[7] For example, a patient may say that he left his glasses at home, bring in a pre-signed check, or pretend to understand rather than risk embarrassment by revealing their comprehension difficulties.[7] Pharmacists should be alert for language comprehension difficulties in patients who ask no questions, bring a friend with them, or those who are persistently noncompliant even with simple instructions.[8]

Patients with difficulties in this area are at risk when dealing with medications in a number of ways.[8] For one thing, they often lack knowledge of basic preventative health care and may be more reliant on self-medication or borrowing other people's medications. There is of course a greater potential for confusing medications at home and of misusing medication because of inability to comprehend the medication label. Difficulties can arise as a result of inability to read or comprehend dosing instructions, labelled warnings regarding expiration dates, and side effects, as well as confusion between look-alike brands. Patients with these difficulties may also be reluctant to ask questions.

Types of Language-Comprehension Difficulties

Pharmacists often encounter difficulties in counseling patients of foreign origin. Comprehension difficulties can include not only language comprehension, but also culturally different ways of expressing and perceiving things.[9] They may have different ways of greetings, different body language (e.g., masking emotions or smiling to conceal grief or anger), and may rely more on nonverbal language for understanding. In addition, different cultures perceive and interpret certain illnesses differently, and describe pain and illness more emotionally or dramatically, or conversely, stoically and nonchalantly. Other differences may include family structure and relationships, religious beliefs and practices, attitudes to food, and attitudes to life events. Most importantly, health beliefs and practices may be different, resulting in use of home remedies, alternative therapies, and certain ways of relating to health-care providers (e.g., blind trust or automatic distrust).

In addition, during discussions with patients, pharmacists often find themselves using jargon, forgetting that many technical pharmaceutical terms are not readily understood by a large percentage of the population. As an example, words such as "void" and "topical" have been reported to be intelligible to only one third of the population, and require a Grade 12 to Grade 13 education level to be understood.[10]

Detection of Poor Language Comprehension

It is important for the pharmacist to realize that many people with language-comprehension difficulties feel embarrassed about their difficulty and often try to hide it. The pharmacist must be tactful in detecting and inquiring about comprehension difficulties, as well as in dealing with those difficulties. At no time should the patient be made to feel that this is a bother to the pharmacist, or that he or she is in any way inferior.

The pharmacist must try to detect the presence and extent of such problems by getting the patient to speak as much as possible during the opening and information-gathering phases of the counseling session. The pharmacist should try to gauge the patient's language level, and reflect this in his own speech. By taking note of the patient's vocabulary during the opening and information-gathering phases of the protocol, the pharmacist may be better able to determine the patient's language-comprehension level. The pharmacist should listen in particular for the words that the patient uses to describe his condition and medication, then use the same words during the counseling session. For example, if the patient says his medication is for "blackouts," then the pharmacist should use this term during counseling rather than terms such as "seizures" or "epilepsy."

Tailoring Counseling to Deal with Language-Comprehension Difficulties

Pharmacists can improve counseling effectiveness with patients exhibiting language-comprehension difficulties by tailoring counseling in a number of ways.

1. *Simplify Explanations.* While avoiding any hint of condescension, the pharmacist should phrase explanations in the simplest terms possible, without sacrificing any necessary information. The patient can be invited to ask the pharmacist questions, and more information can then be provided at the patient's request.

2. *Avoid Difficult Words.* Some alternate words for difficult or specialized words often used in patient counseling are suggested in Table 8.1. In addition, general phrases such as "plenty of water" and "on an empty stomach" have been found to lead to confusion and should be explained more precisely by the pharmacist.[11]

3. *Involve Family.* Where necessary (and where possible), a family member or other individual should be enlisted as an interpreter. If this is done, the pharmacist should see the patient and interpreter together and ask that the discussion be translated in sections so that the patient can be involved and so that patient queries can be responded to. This way the pharmacist can be sure that the information was actually transmitted to the patient and that any misunderstandings or concerns of the patient were dealt with.

4. *Use Various Counseling Methods and Aids.* The use of diagrams and pictures is also helpful where there are language-comprehension difficulties. In addition, some computer programs for pharmacy include translations of prescription-label directions into other languages. However, the pharmacist, or, at least, pharmacy personnel, should be able to understand these instructions so that errors can be detected. The United States Pharmacopeia (USP) has also developed supplemental labels with graphic illustrations of common directions.[7]

5. *Obtain Feedback.* Obtaining feedback from patients concerning their understanding is particularly important for patients with language-comprehension difficulties. The pharmacist should solicit feedback from the patient at several points during the counseling session to ensure that the patient fully understands what he or she has heard. To evaluate the effectiveness of the counseling, the pharmacist may ask the patient, directly or through the translator, to repeat back instructions, and may ask if the patient has any concerns or questions.

6. *Follow-up.* As well, follow-up contact with the patient or family members the next day and possibly regularly over the following weeks can be important in ensuring that the patient has understood.

Table 8.1   Alternatives to Difficult Words

analgesic	*to help stop pain*
topically	*on the skin*
contraceptive	*birth control*
coronary thrombosis	*heart attack*
discoloration	*change in color*
dyspepsia	*indigestion*
gastrointestinal	*stomach or digestive system*
over the counter	*medicine you buy without a prescription*
embolism	*blood clot*
therapy	*treatment*
completion	*end, finish*
decrease	*lower*
diagnosis	*problem, condition*
diminish	*get less, slow down*
elevate	*raise*
eliminate	*get rid of*
excessive	*too much*
sensation	*feeling*
severity	*how bad*
termination	*end*
utilize	*use*

Adapted from Hilts L, Krilyk BJ. W.R.I.T.E. Write readable information to educate. Hamilton, Canada, 1991. Hamilton Civic Hospitals, Hamilton General Division, Chedoke-McMaster Hospitals.

Counseling Patients with Disabilities

Various disabilities that patients may have can also cause difficulties during patient counseling.

Detecting Disabilities

The pharmacist should note at the start of the encounter whether the patient has any apparent disabilities. Sometimes, however, disabilities may not be detectable at the beginning, but may become apparent during counseling. For example, a patient with hearing difficulties may respond inappropriately to questions; turn his head so that his ear faces the pharmacist; make gestures to indicate that he is having difficulty hearing (cupping a hand behind an ear); make frequent requests for repetition; look around for the speaker; use loud speech; or omit word endings such as t, s, sh, f, and v.[12,13]

One difficulty identified by pharmacists in dealing with disabled patients is making inaccurate judgments about them, particularly regarding their intellect and personalities.[1] The pharmacist must be tactful in detecting and inquiring about physical disabilities, and every effort should be made to make the patient feel comfortable and in no way inferior. Physical disabilities should *not* be associated with mental disabilities. Therefore, patronizing actions such as addressing the patient with slow speech, loud voice, or extravagant praise should be avoided.[14] Alternatively, neither the patient's disabilities nor the patient himself should be ignored.

Tailoring Counseling to Deal with Disabled Patients

Pharmacists can improve counseling effectiveness with disabled patients by tailoring the counseling session in a number of ways:

1. *Be Prepared for Feelings.* Pharmacists need to be prepared for the feelings that dealing with the disabled patient may arouse in themselves and other staff such as embarrassment, aversion, pity, and dread.[14] In addition, the frustrations with their disabilities, and irritation with others' attitudes can cause the disabled patient to react aggressively or uncooperatively.[14] If pharmacists are prepared, they can make an attempt to control such feelings in themselves and make allowances for such feelings in others.

2. *Offer Assistance.* Assistance should be offered where the need is obvious or when the patient requests it, rather than automatically provided.[5] The patient should be asked what he would like done, and how it can be accomplished. For example, the patient should be asked how he prefers to be helped up the steps rather than just having his arm grabbed. The pharmacist should address the patient directly, rather than speaking to his attendant or relative. Direct vocal and eye contact should be made.

3. *Allow Extra Time.* Extra time should be allowed for counseling the disabled patient. Time may need to be allowed for physical needs (e.g., maneuvering a wheelchair into a counseling area); the patient's slower speech; or the use of communication aids (e.g., pointing to words and letters on a word board). Silence should be tolerated (for up to 20 to 30 seconds) to allow the patient to collect his thoughts and to prepare a response.[13] The pharmacist should simply wait quietly or cue the patient visually to indicate that the patient should continue. Of course, prolonged silence indicates communication breakdown.

4. *Dealing with Hearing Problems.* To compensate for a patient's hearing problem, the pharmacist should not yell, but rather should try to enunciate clearly and face the person directly, with the light facing the pharmacist.[5,12,13] Use of simple sentences and familiar vocabulary will facilitate lip reading.[5,12,13] The pharmacist might also supplement verbal explanations with written notes, print materials, or charts and diagrams. In cases of total deafness, a family member or caregiver who knows sign language may be able to provide assistance.

5. *Dealing with Vision Problems.* For patients with severe loss of vision, the pharmacist should identify himself and any other people who are with him, using people's names to clarify to whom the conversation is being directed.[5] Medication bottles and containers can be varied in size to help identification of different medications, and bright-colored stickers can be used to assist patients with limited vision.

6. *Emphasize Nonverbal Communication.* Nonverbal communication is also important when dealing with disabled patients such as facing the patient, inclining the body towards the patient, or holding the patient's hand. Such gestures can make the patient feel more comfortable and send the message that the pharmacist is interested in the patient. These nonverbal actions also cue the patient that the pharmacist is about to speak.[13] Although it is expected by the disabled that people may take a second look, staring for long periods is inappropriate, as is avoidance of eye contact altogether.

7. *Attend to the Environment.* Preferably the counseling environment should be quiet and well lighted. The pharmacist should be positioned as close to the patient as possible for comfort, on the same level (e.g., the pharmacist should sit or squat down to the patient's level when speaking to a patient in a wheelchair). The pharmacy and counseling area should be accessible by wheelchairs, and barriers such as boxes or extra furniture should be kept clear of walk ways. Products and patient-information materials should be reachable from a wheelchair, and staff should be alerted to provide patients with assistance where it appears necessary. Decals and signs should be used in the pharmacy window to indicate that it is wheelchair accessible.[5]

8. *Involve the Patient and Solicit Feedback.* As discussed regarding patients' language difficulties, efforts should be made to ensure that the patient is involved as much as possible in the patient-counseling discussion. Every effort should be made to assess the patient's understanding and to respond to his or her concerns by soliciting feedback during patient counseling, and by arranging for follow-up contacts.

9. *Learn More About the Disabled in Your Community.* Pharmacists can learn more about how to improve communication with the disabled patients in their community by contacting local chapters of organizations serving the disabled, such as the national Spinal Cord Injury Associa-

tion, the Muscular Dystrophy Association, the Multiple Sclerosis Society, United Cerebral Palsy; the Easter Seal Society; the United Ostomy Association, etc.[5]

Counseling Patients on Medication Requiring Administration or Complicated Instructions

Many medications have complicated instruction or require instruction in administration. Pharmacists can improve counseling effectiveness in these situations by tailoring counseling in a number of ways.

1. *Use Appropriate Counseling Methods and Aids.* If the patient's medication requires special application or administration, the pharmacist should demonstrate the use of the apparatus in question. A videotape might be used in place of a personal demonstration. It is also helpful to provide written instructions that include a diagram of the procedure.

   The patient should be given the opportunity to practice the procedure during the counseling session, enabling the patient and the pharmacist to identify any problems or concerns.

   Where complicated instructions are involved, the pharmacist should also provide supplementary written instructions, medication charts, or memory aids such as pill-reminder containers to simplify the process as much as possible, as discussed in Chapter 6 .

2. *Solicit Feedback.* It is especially important in these situations for the pharmacist to obtain feedback from the patient regarding his or her understanding of the instructions. The patient should be asked to tell the pharmacist how he or she intends to take the medication after the pharmacist has explained. The patient should also be asked to practice with the pharmacist observing. Tact should be used to make sure the patient doesn't feel foolish repeating back or revealing lack of understanding. For example, the pharmacist may say, "Just so that I'm sure that I have explained things well enough, please tell me, in your own words, how you will use this medication." This puts the responsibility on the pharmacist rather than the patient for any lack of understanding.

3. *Follow-up.* Since patients may forget complicated instructions or run into difficulties after they have returned home, follow-up is important. In addition, when the patient returns to the pharmacy for a refill of the medication, counseling should involve finding out in detail how the patient has been using the medication. The patient should be asked to demonstrate the use of medication so that the pharmacist can detect any problems with the patient's technique.

Counseling Patients with Conditions that May Arouse Emotions

Certain medical conditions can arouse unpleasant emotions in a patient, and patients may be particularly worried, embarrassed, or defensive about their conditions. Although any condition could arouse these emotions, certain conditions have a particular social stigma, poor prognosis, or implications of life-long effects. Conditions that may present particular difficulty in counseling include psychiatric illnesses, epilepsy, diabetes, and conditions that may be fatal, such as cancer and AIDS-related conditions. In these conditions, the patient's lifestyle is often significantly affected by the condition. In addition, the patient must come to terms with a possibly life-long condition that may not improve or may worsen. The patient may also have to deal with extensive treatment programs that have significant side effects, as well as complicated administration.

Tailoring Counseling to Deal with Patients with Difficult Conditions

When dealing with patients with these difficult conditions, it is particularly important for the pharmacist to be tactful in discussing the condition, being careful to use the patient's own terms. In addition, the pharmacist must deal with his or her own biases and fears regarding the condition that may cause her to avoid discussion or to offer false reassurance. Counseling in these situations can be most effective by tailoring counseling in a number of ways.

1. *Identify the Patient's Needs.* When dealing with patients with difficult conditions, it is important to spend time initially determining the patient's needs. The patient's understanding of the condition, as well as his or her attitudes to treatment are important to ascertain, particularly concerning the patient's willingness to participate in the treatment.[15] Detailed questions should be asked in this regard, and an assessment form should be used to assist the pharmacist in asking specific questions related to the patient's condition.[15]

    Documentation by the pharmacist of the patient's needs at the first counseling session and at follow-up sessions will help the pharmacist to track particular concerns and take appropriate action.

2. *Help Patient Make Adjustments to Daily Life.* Since these conditions are long-term and require many adjustments to the patient's life, pharmacists should pay particular attention to helping patients to integrate medication use into their daily lives. In addition, monitoring for effectiveness and side effects could be assisted through use of a log book for the patient to record daily occurrences, as well as through attentive follow-up by the pharmacist at repeat visits as well as in between through arranged follow-up telephone calls.

    Due to the complexity of regimens for many of these conditions, the pharmacist should assist the patient in organizing and remembering doses, as well as, where possible, making recommendations to the physician for simplifying regimens.[16]

3. *Assist the Patient to Use Appropriate Terminology.* When discussing the condition, the pharmacist should review common terminology for the condition with the patient. Since other health-care providers will likely use these terms, this will assist the patient to participate in discussions.

4. *Encourage Participation by the Patient in His or Her Treatment.* Participation by the patient is particularly important, since treatment will be on-going. The patient should be encouraged to suggest changes according to his or her own needs, and to take responsibility for his or her treatment as much as possible. This will increase the patient's feelings of self-worth and make him or her more psychologically able to deal with other aspects of the condition.

5. *Solicit Feedback.* Again, feedback is important to make sure there are no misunderstandings between the pharmacist and the patient.[16]

6. *Provide Additional Motivational Counseling.* Due to the long duration of treatment, the patient will need additional motivational counseling. More supervision, use of compliance aids, changes to reduce or eliminate side effects, goal-setting, and improvements in the patient–clinician relationship may be used to enhance the motivation of these patients.[15,16] On-going reinforcement and support will also be needed through follow-up.

7. *Provide Privacy.* Providing privacy is particularly important for counseling these patients, since discussions likely involve the patient's feelings and concerns about his or her condition and treatment.

8. *Special Considerations for Terminally Ill Patients.* As discussed in Chapter 3, dying patients often go through various stages of emotions (denial, anger, bargaining, depression, and acceptance). Suggestions were made in Chapter 3 for ways that pharmacists can help the patient during each stage. The following suggestions are also helpful[17,18]:
   - Be as relaxed as possible;
   - Show genuine concern and care;
   - Use listening skills as well as nonverbal communication to let the patient know you are interested as well as to encourage the patient to express his or her own feelings;
   - Allow silence;
   - Be prepared to defer counseling to another time if the patient does not feel well enough;
   - Help the patient to make choices;
   - Do not tell the patient how he should feel or that you know how he feels;
   - Do not try to talk the patient out of feeling angry, depressed, sad, etc.;
   - Be as honest as possible.

Counseling Elderly Patients

Elderly patients comprise a growing segment of the pharmacist's clientele. As mentioned earlier, the elderly in no way form a homogeneous group. They vary greatly, not only in their physical and mental capacities, but also in their financial circumstances and personal wants and needs. The number of illness conditions and medications used tends to increase with age, so that there may be great variations between 60-year-old and 90-year-old patients (all considered "elderly"), but there may also be great differences between individuals. As a result, each patient should be considered on an individual basis. There are, however, various considerations that should be made in counseling this group of patients in general.

Difficulties in Counseling the Elderly

Elderly patients use more prescriptions than any other group of patients. Although people over 65 years of age comprise 12% of the general population, they use 30% of all prescription drugs.[19] They also experience an increased incidence of illness, particularly chronic illnesses; 80% of people over 65 years of age reports at least one chronic ailment. Since aging is accompanied by various changes in physiology, the pharmacokinetics of many drugs are different, resulting in an increased risk of adverse reactions in the elderly, nearly double that of younger adults.[13,19]

Another consideration in counseling the elderly patient involves various barriers to communication.[20] One barrier is the attitude of the pharmacist. Younger pharmacists in particular may have difficulty in understanding an elderly patient's point of view, the effects of history and experiences on their attitudes and ways of behaving that have become rigid over time and experience. The pharmacist must also overcome the feelings aroused regarding his or her own aging, such as anxiety about changing appearance, infirmity, dependence, and death.[20]

Pharmacists may also not fully recognize the elderly patient's limitations and the effect of several disabilities compounded. These include physical disabilities as discussed above such as hearing loss (experienced by 60% of the elderly) and vision impairment even with corrective lenses (experienced by 20% of the elderly). Other disabilities experienced by the elderly include dementia, language disorders resulting often from stroke (dysarthria, dysphasia), difficulties eating because of dental problems, altered pain threshold, transportation difficulties, diminished personal economic resources, loss of physical energy, and isolation.[13,20,21]

In addition, elderly patients have been found to have more difficulty than younger patients in distinguishing between tablets of similar size, shape, and color.[11]

Tailoring Counseling to Deal with Difficulties in Counseling the Elderly

In considering how to approach counseling the elderly, it is worthwhile considering what older patients say they want from their pharmacists. In a recent survey, elderly patients were found to be quite loyal customers (three out of five said they use only one pharmacy regularly) and generally satisfied with their pharmacies.[22] Although low costs were at the top of their wish lists, the elderly also reported wanting quality of care, information from the pharmacist, and friendliness. In another survey, elderly patients were more willing than other age groups to pay for information services from the pharmacist.[23]

There are a number of ways that pharmacists can tailor counseling to deal more effectively with the elderly.

1. *Recognize Feelings.* In order to effectively counsel elderly patients, the pharmacist must first face his own feelings regarding aging. One suggestion is to remember that the elderly patient has not always been old.[20] The pharmacist should ask himself, "What was this person like when he or she was my age? When was that? What was going on in the world then? What has happened in the intervening years?"[20] In this way, the pharmacist might better understand what the patient's difficulties are today, particularly if he or she spends a few minutes actually discussing some of these questions with the patient before getting down to the details of the medication counseling.[20]

2. *Attend to Drug-Use Problems.* As a result of the greater risks of the elderly experiencing drug use problems, patient counseling for elderly patients should involve detailed discussion of potential adverse effects. This should include information regarding ways to identify adverse effects, ways to reduce the chance of occurrence, what to do if they occur, how to modify the effects, and when to report to the physician immediately.

3. *Provide Time.* To address the elderly patients' counseling needs and wants, pharmacists should be prepared to spend time in the initial phase of the counseling making the patient comfortable, discussing general topics as desired by the patient. This not only helps the pharmacists–patient relationship (particularly for lonely, isolated patients) but also allows the pharmacist to evaluate the patient's difficulties that may potentially interfere with medication use as mentioned above.

4. *Deal with Disabilities.* If disabilities are identified, the pharmacist should make sure that the techniques discussed above for dealing with the disabled are used. In addition, if memory problems or dementia of any type is suspected, the patient should be asked if other family members or caregivers can be contacted to reinforce medication information. It may also be necessary for the pharmacist to discuss concerns with the patient's physician, as this may be the first indication of problems.

5. *Consider Patients' Specific Needs.* Dosing schedules should be discussed with the elderly patient to take into consideration changing habits of the elderly such as changes in eating or sleeping patterns (e.g., napping in the afternoon).[21] Difficulties discussed above regarding difficulties in counseling patients with chronic conditions should also be taken into consideration.

6. *Provide Follow-up.* For patients who live alone, careful monitoring is important, and follow-up contact arrangements should be made.

7. *Provide Privacy.* Privacy should also be considered, since the elderly often become embarrassed at sharing personal information. [23]

8. *Emphasize Compliance.* In a review of studies of drug use by the elderly, Green and colleagues found that, in spite of all the difficulties faced by the elderly, there is no evidence to conclude that the elderly are more noncompliant than younger patients.[24] However, since the need of the elderly to be compliant is particularly critical given the seriousness of many of their conditions, the pharmacist should tailor counseling to put some emphasis on ensuring compliance.

9. *Select Appropriate Counseling Methods and Aids.* When selecting the method of information provision to elderly patients, pharmacists should consider patients' disabilities and provide material that they can easily use (e.g., large print labels, etc). In addition, elderly patients reportedly like written information to take home and peruse at their own pace, or possibly to review with another caregiver.

   Studies of different education strategies used for the elderly have concluded that drug knowledge is most likely to be improved by providing small amounts of specific information, and by a combination of a reminder aid with oral reinforcement.[25,26]

Many drug-education programs have been planned particularly for the elderly. The concept of the "brown bag" clinic has been developed and is used in many communities across the country. Kits are available to assist pharmacists in conducting these clinics from The National Council of Patient Information and Education (see Appendix A). Perhaps the strength of this program is that it allows for individual assessment of each elderly patient. Other resources available for counseling the elderly are also listed in Appendix A.

Interference During Patient Counseling

Another difficulty for pharmacists in patient counseling involves interruptions. The counseling protocol may be interrupted in a number of ways, by patients as well as by other individuals requiring the pharmacist's attention.

Dealing with Outside Interruptions

Interruptions during counseling by staff, other patients, sales representatives, and telephone calls are all a fact of life for many pharmacists. The pharmacy environment, in general, allows for interruptions, and this can be very difficult for the pharmacist and patient to deal with. The need for privacy in patient counseling has been mentioned earlier, in relation to the needs of the patient; however, the pharmacist also needs to have some privacy in order to focus on the patient.

In addition to securing a relatively private place to conduct patient counseling, the pharmacist should organize his or her activities so that there should be no need for interruptions (e.g., sales representatives are seen by appointment, telephone-answering procedures are clearly set down) and strict instructions should be given as to the circumstances under which interruptions may be tolerated.

Dealing with Interruption by the Patient

Although patient involvement in counseling should be encouraged, patients sometimes ask questions or make comments that do not relate specifically to the topic under discussion. Although the pharmacist should encourage the patient to talk, and spontaneity should be encouraged, it is the pharmacist's responsibility to keep the conversation relevant and maintain control of the interview at all times.[27] In general, the pharmacist should try to follow the counseling protocol, resuming after an interruption, rather than altering the order of counseling according the patient's comments. This will minimize the chance of omitting important information or creating confusion.

If a patient's question is related in some way to the medication or condition that is the subject of the counseling, of course the question should be addressed immediately, at least partially, with a suggestion that it be discussed more fully later on, if necessary. If, for example, during the opening phase of the session, the patient mentions that he will be going to a party and asks if he may drink alcohol with the medication, the pharmacist can comment briefly that this would not be a good idea, then suggest that he will return to the subject later on in the counseling session. The pharmacist could resume the protocol of information gathering, then discuss alcohol use further, including suggested methods for dealing with situations like parties, during the information-giving phase.

If, on the other hand, the patient's question is totally unrelated to the topic of the counseling, the pharmacist could acknowledge the question and politely defer it until after the present counseling session. For example, if the patient asks a question about the currently advertised sale in the pharmacy, the pharmacist could acknowledge that there is a sale and say that he would be happy to ask a clerk to show the patient the sale products after they have finished their discussion.

Counseling to Overcome Emotional Situations and Conflict

Pharmacists must sometimes deal with patient-counseling situations that are particularly difficult, because there is a strong emotional element or an element of conflict. The source of the conflict is usually a difference in opinion between the pharmacist and patient, such as a patient's complaint about a particular product. A patient's strong emotions may be a result of the pharmacist's actions or for a reason unrelated to the pharmacist, such as extreme worry about illness or medication use, or emotional upset for any number of personal reasons. In addition, pharmacists should realize that patients are often in physical discomfort. When people have these kinds of feelings, they often react with strong emotions like anger, or appear distraught and depressed, sometimes tearful. Consider the following situation involving conflict.

Counseling Situation

Mr. Williams is a middle-aged executive who has been waiting in the pharmacy for a refill of his cimetidine 600-mg prescription. It is now ready and the pharmacist calls him to the pharmacy counter.

Pharmacist: Hello, Mr. Williams. Your prescription is ready for you now. I'll just spend a few minutes to discuss it with you to make sure you're getting the most benefit from it.

Patient: *(looking and sounding aggravated)* It's about time! I've been waiting here half my lunch hour, and I think it's ridiculous! I'm a busy person, and I simply don't have the time...

Pharmacist: *(ignoring the patient's comments and cutting in)* Well, it's ready now. I see you've been taking the cimetidine for a few months now. How have you been taking it?

Patient: *(still fuming)* Twice a day, just as it says on the label.

Pharmacist: *(ignoring the patient's obvious anger)* Good. And how have you been feeling?

Patient: *(raising his voice more)* Just fine, until I had to come in here and get the run around. I think...

Pharmacist: *(cutting in)* Well, we've been very busy today. If you'd phoned 24 hours ahead as it says on the label...

Patient: *(cutting in, almost yelling)* I phoned ahead like it says on the label, and it still wasn't ready.

Pharmacist: *(sounding a little unsure)* Oh, well, I wasn't here yesterday. They probably had to call the doctor.

Patient: *(still sounding angry)* Why do they have to do that? She knows I need this stuff.

Pharmacist: *(more sure of herself now, authoritative tone)* Legally we need to contact the doctor to refill prescriptions.

Patient: *(yelling, attracting the attention of other waiting patients)* I don't care about your laws. I'm supposed to be on this all the time, and the doctor said I could get it whenever I wanted.

Pharmacist: Oh, well, I don't know anything about that. I just came on duty a few minutes ago. The other pharmacist must have handled it.

Patient: Sure, just pass the buck. That's always the way with you people. You just put in your time and don't give a hoot about what's going on.

Pharmacist: *(angry now, raising her voice)* What do you mean "you people?" I'm a very responsible pharmacist. You have no right to say that about me!

Patient: *(giving up, still yelling)* Just give me my prescription and let me get out of here! And I won't be back, that's for sure!

Pharmacist: *(practically throwing the prescription at the patient)* Fine! Here! *(Patient walks away angrily, commenting to other waiting patients as he passes about the inefficiency of this pharmacy)*

Discussion

This patient probably won't come back to the pharmacy. More importantly, the pharmacist was not able to discuss the medication, and therefore, didn't have a chance to discover that the patient was experiencing some dizziness, causing him to skip doses on days when he has important meetings. In addition, the patient didn't have the opportunity to ask whether he could have a drink at a party he planned to attend that evening. Finally, both the patient and the pharmacist left the situation feeling stressed.

In such situations, the pharmacist's first instinct may be to avoid the issue, for his or her sake or the patient's comfort. If the counseling is to proceed, however, the patient's emotions or the source of conflict must be dealt with first. Strong emotions will distract the patient from participating, making it difficult for the pharmacist to gather information and for the patient, in a turbulent state of mind, to learn anything about his or her medication. By trying to resolve the situation, the pharmacist might even discover important information pertaining to medication use.

The techniques for dealing with these difficult situations involve using many of the communication techniques discussed in Chapter 7. The most important elements in handling such situations are to recognize the patient's feelings and concerns and, if at all possible, to discuss them. The emphasis during the counseling session should be placed on resolving the patient's concerns and calming strong emotions. Specific suggestions for tailoring counseling to deal with difficult situations will follow, and are summarized in Table 8.2.

Remaining in Control of Personal Emotions

When presented with an emotional patient or a conflict, the pharmacist must deal with his or her own emotions as well as the patient's, resulting in interpersonal stress.[28] The most common causes of interpersonal stress for pharmacists include commands given by others, anger directed to the pharmacist, criticism, inattentiveness by another individual (not listening, ignoring, avoiding eye contact), impulsive behavior by another, and making mistakes.[28] The resulting emotions may be anger, frustration, embarrassment, disgust, or general discomfort about the topic under discussion.

To deal with difficult situations, the pharmacist should be prepared for such feelings. By recognizing and accepting these feelings (rather than trying to deny them), the pharmacist will be better able to control such emotions and maintain a detached and nonjudgmental attitude with the patient. This by no means implies that pharmacists should remain cold or unfeeling; on the contrary, it suggests that, by becoming familiar with her own responses, the pharmacist will be better equipped to maintain a professional demeanor and to help the patient deal with his emotions. Responding with an emotional outburst is invariably counter-productive.

One technique for dealing with interpersonal stress is desensitization.[28] This is a technique whereby the pharmacist gradually makes himself "less sensitive" to a stressor. It involves being exposed to the stressor for increasing lengths of time until the pharmacist "learns to put up with it." This often occurs over time as pharmacists gain experience in dealing with patients. However, a more painless and quicker way is to actively pursue desensitization through a relaxation exercise in which the pharmacist imagines the stressful situation in detail for 5 seconds at a time, then imagines a peaceful, relaxing scene.[28] This is repeated several times, increasing the length of time of imagining the stressor by 10 seconds each time. This whole process is repeated several times a day for several days until the pharmacist feels comfortable with the situation.

Another technique involves the pharmacist saying positive coping statements to himself, while the situation is occurring. Such statements may be: "I can handle this"; "I can cope with this"; "It's not so terrible"; "I can stand it"; "Everything's going to be all right"[28] These can also be more specific to the situation, for example, "Stay calm"; "He doesn't really mean it personally"; "He isn't feeling well"; etc.

A third technique is covert rehearsal, whereby the pharmacist imagines himself successfully coping with the stressor.[28] As with desensitization, the pharmacist imagines a situation that he generally finds difficult. Then, he imagines going through the situation, what he might say, perhaps imagining the surroundings and how the patient is behaving, but imagining that things work out and that the patient responds to his statements. (More details about these technique and practise exercises are provided by Gerrard and colleagues.[28])

Other techniques useful for coping in such situations include visualizing that the situation is over, distracting oneself with activities such as doodling (as long as it is out of sight of the patient), and simply not responding to personal criticism or insults from the patient, since they are often designed simply to put the pharmacist at a disadvantage.

Letting Patients Vent Their Feelings
The scientific training that pharmacists have received will have taught them to be analytical in their problem-solving approaches. As a result, they may tend to focus on the problem rather than on the patient. As discussed in the previous chapter, pharmacists often tend to deal with situations by asking questions and making judgments or giving advice. This, however, removes the focus from the patient and may result in an angry response. It is more effective, particularly in difficult situations for the pharmacist to focus on the patient.

The pharmacist should start by giving the patient an opportunity to vent his or her feelings. By passively listening, the pharmacist will allow the patient to get his or her concerns, or any emotions, out in the open and possibly to calm down a little.[29] If the patient is very distraught, and possibly even in tears, he should be allowed to sit quietly, preferably in privacy, while he regains control. If the patient is extremely upset and unable to regain self-control, it may be necessary to defer medication counseling to a later time, to be conducted either on the telephone or in person.

Show Empathy for the Patient
As discussed in Chapter 7, showing empathy is an important part of patient counseling, and this is particularly true in difficult situations.[30] After the patient

has had his say, the pharmacist should show empathy for his situation. Rather than arguing, becoming defensive, or jumping to give advice, the pharmacist can encourage the patient to discuss his problems and complaints through active listening. This allows the patient to clarify what is bothering him, and it helps the pharmacist to better understand the situation (e.g., the patient isn't actually angry at the pharmacist but frustrated with his doctor).

Probe to Clarify the Problem

The fourth step in dealing with difficult situations will in some cases involve probing to make clear more details about the problem. As discussed in the previous chapter, probing requires a certain degree of skill to avoid causing the patient to become defensive or impatient. Again, this not only helps the pharmacist to get a better grasp of the problem, but also helps to focus and calm the patient.

Provide Explanations and Suggestions

Once the pharmacist has a grasp of the problem, she may need to offer the patient an explanation or simply provide some information. The patient's point of view, not the pharmacist's, should always direct the pharmacist's explanations. For example, when explaining that a prescription cannot be refilled without the doctor's authorization, rather than simply stating pharmacy law, the pharmacist should explain that it is in the patient's interest that the physician be apprised of the situation.

Where possible, suggestions should also be offered to help solve the problem. Several alternatives should be offered where possible, so that the patient can maintain a feeling of choice, and hence, can feel more in control of the situation. Recall from Chapter 3 that patients often feel a lack of control because of their condition and treatment in the health-care process, which often results in frustration, anger or feelings of hopelessness. By allowing the patient to make some decisions, the pharmacist can improve the patient's feelings of self-worth and control.

If the reason for the patient's distress involves an error on the pharmacist's part or some sort of misunderstanding, the pharmacist should acknowledge the error, sincerely apologize, and offer a remedy where appropriate.[30] It's best to avoid making excuses or "passing the buck." Even if the pharmacist dealing with the situation is not personally responsible for the problem (e.g., if another pharmacist originally dealt with the patient), he or she should still accept the responsibility of dealing with it. If, however, the patient demands to speak with someone else, this should be politely arranged.

Provide Privacy

Because most of these situations are quite sensitive, the pharmacist should provide privacy, if possible. If necessary, the discussion should be continued later, by telephone. This allows both the pharmacist and the patient to be more comfortable in the discussion, as well as preventing others from becoming involved (e.g., another nearby customer entering into a disagreement about pricing).

Be Assertive

Assertiveness on the pharmacist's part is also important in dealing with conflict and emotional situations.[30] It can help to resolve the situation in such a way that neither party ends up the "loser." If the situation cannot be resolved because outside input is necessary or because the patient is too upset to continue, assertiveness is critical. The pharmacist may simply have to stand his ground and end the situation.

Although the patient's point of view should be considered first, the pharmacist can ask the patient to consider the pharmacist's own point of view later in the discussion. She may also state her feelings, for example, "I feel very embarrassed about this."

Provide Positive Messages to the Patient

Positive messages, both verbal and nonverbal, will help to calm a situation and improve the interaction. Such things as using the patient's name, smiling, giving the patient full attention and honest recognition, apologizing for any inconvenience caused by the pharmacist or pharmacy all help to provide a positive message. In addition, comments should be phrased in a positive light. For example, rather than, "I can't help you," the pharmacist should say, "I'd like to help you. I just need a little more information."

End the Situation on a Positive Note

Finally, whenever possible, the pharmacist should attempt to end the situation on a positive note, perhaps by recapping a positive solution, or by reiterating what has been tried to resolve the situation. The pharmacist might also suggest some sort of follow-up, such as asking the patient to telephone to discuss the outcome of suggested measures, or offering to call the patient.

Sometimes, situations involving distressed or upset patients cannot be resolved at the time. It may be necessary for the pharmacist to end the encounter if the patient is unable to regain control, or if the session threatens to become too lengthy. Assertiveness on the pharmacist's part may be needed here to summarize the situation, and bring it to a close. Arrangements might be made for further discussion or for the patient to seek other help. A statement might be made to curtail the situation, such as, "I'm sorry I'm not able to help you any further today. I've tried to explain the situation to you and offered some suggestions. Perhaps we can discuss this further when you're feeling calmer." The pharmacist can then use nonverbal language to indicate that the discussion is over (e.g., turning her body to begin walking away, making eye contact with the next patient, stapling the prescription bag, etc).

Table 8.2 Process for Dealing with Emotional Situations and Conflict

Remain in control of personal emotions

Let the patient vent his or her feelings

Show empathy for the patient

Probe to clarify the problem

Provide explanations and suggestions

Provide privacy

Be assertive

Provide positive messages to the patient

End the situation on a positive note

When the pharmacist uses these techniques, the counseling situation with Mr. Williams ends differently.

Alternate Counseling Situation

<u>Pharmacist</u>: Hello, Mr. Williams. Your prescription is ready for you now. I'll just spend a few minutes to discuss it with you to make sure you're getting the most benefit from it.

<u>Patient</u>: *(looking and sounding aggravated)* It's about time! I've been waiting here half my lunch hour, and I think that's ridiculous! I'm a busy person, and I simply don't have the time to stand around and wait in this pharmacy.

<u>Pharmacist</u>: *(listens and waits for patient to finish speaking, empathetic tone)* Let's step over to the counseling area to talk. *(leads the way to the counseling booth)* I can see that you're upset about having to wait, and I can understand why that would annoy you. I'm sorry if you were inconvenienced.

<u>Patient</u>: *(calmer but still fuming)* Well, why wasn't it ready?

<u>Pharmacist</u>: *(empathetic tone)* I know it may seem like a long time to get your prescription ready, but we did need to contact the doctor, to...

<u>Patient</u>: *(cutting in angrily)* Why did you have to do that? She knows I need this stuff.

<u>Pharmacist</u>: *(calmly)* That may be so, but she also likes to be kept informed of how often you need your medication, so she can know how your condition is and whether the medication is helping.

<u>Patient</u>: *(calmer)* Oh, I guess that's true, but I thought I had refills on this prescription.

<u>Pharmacist</u>: *(sounding confident)* I'll check on that for you. I wasn't here at the time it was processed.

Patient: *(still a little angry)* Sure, just pass the buck. That's always the way with you people. You just put in your time and don't give a hoot about what's going on.

Pharmacist: *(controlling her anger and speaking in a calm voice)* It may sound like I'm passing the buck, but I'm just trying to explain why I wasn't sure about the refill order. Again, I'm sorry if you're upset.

Patient: *(calming down and feeling sorry for insulting the pharmacist)* OK. I shouldn't have become so worked up. That's my problem, and probably why I need these pills. I've got a big case I'm working on, and I guess I'm on edge.

Pharmacist: *(smiling, empathetic tone)* That's OK. It sounds like you're really under stress. Let's just slow down for a few minutes, and I'll go over your prescription to make sure you're getting the most benefit from it. It'll just take a few minutes and then you'll have some time left to relax before heading back to your work.

Patient: *(smiling back)* OK. I wanted to ask you about drinking with this medication...*(Patient and pharmacist proceed to discuss the medication. The pharmacist identifies the patient's medication-related problems, then counsels him regarding alcohol use, dealing with dizziness, and the need for compliance. She also checks the patient file and confirms that there were no authorized refills and explains to the patient that his prescription will be ready for him next time if he allows a full 24 to 48 hours for the pharmacist to contact the physician.)*

Discussion

This time the pharmacist responded right away to the patient's anger. She listened passively until he was finished speaking, then suggested they move to a more private area to avoid other patients overhearing. She responded empathetically and then tried to explain what had happened. Her explanation did not cite the law, but used optimal control of therapy as the reason for having to call the doctor. She did not let herself get angry, but remained assertive, letting the patient see her point of view. Her smile, calm voice, and empathy for the patient allowed the counseling to maintain a positive note. Having dealt with the patient's anger first, she was then able to proceed with counseling the patient effectively.

Issues Involving Drug-Product Selection

Federal and state laws allow (some require) pharmacists to substitute a generic drug product for a brand-name drug product that has been prescribed unless the prescriber or patient state that substitution is not to take place.[31] In addition, many private and state drug plans have adopted a "positive formulary," which lists therapeutically equivalent or interchangeable drug products that the pharmacist may dispense (or in some cases is required to dispense); or alternatively a "negative formulary," which lists drug products that are not therapeutically equivalent and may not be interchanged.[31,32] As well as substituting products because they are bound to, pharmacists may also suggest to patients, and where necessary to the physician, that a chemically or therapeutically equivalent product be substituted in order to reduce costs.

It is understood in this discussion that before a product is substituted, the pharmacist will evaluate the clinical aspects of the situation. This should include consideration of the patient's sensitivities to inactive ingredients and the patient's previous use of the product.

As a result, pharmacists from time to time fill prescriptions with products that, although considered equivalent (either chemically or therapeutically), are made by a different manufacturer to that which the physician ordered, or to that which the patient received previously. In most states, pharmacists are required to notify or inform the patient of the substitution.[31]

By providing appropriately timed and carefully worded information, the pharmacist can often avoid future problems. For example, patients receiving a substituted prescription who have not been informed may notice that their medication is a different brand to that named by the physician. They may hear other people's concerns about substitution after they have taken their prescription home. They may then become concerned and either become noncompliant or return to the pharmacist and angrily demand an explanation. Rather than wait for this situation to occur, the pharmacist should discuss substitution with a patient at the time of dispensing, whether or not he or she is required by law to do this.

There are a number of additional issues that pharmacists should be aware of and should be prepared to discuss with patients. Of course, individual pharmacists may have personal views regarding some of these issues, and some retail pharmacy companies may have store policies regarding the handling of such issues. This discussion in no way intends to dictate a particular view, and pharmacists must make decisions based on their own judgment.

First, the pharmacist should explain to the patient the reason for the substitution (e.g., to be covered by the third-party plan or to reduce the prescription price to the patient). In addition, the pharmacist should explain the equivalency of the prescribed and substituted products. Such an explanation may include the approval of substitution by the state and the FDA and the listing of equivalent products in a formulary. Pharmacists may have their own views about these issues, but they should attempt to provide accurate and unbiased information to patients. In addition, it is advisable to avoid causing the patient undue alarm.

Patients often hear the terms "generic" and "brand name" in the media or referred to by pharmacists, but are unclear or confused about their meanings. The pharmacist may realize that there is a misunderstanding in this regard, or the patient may directly ask the pharmacist what these terms mean. It is therefore necessary for the pharmacist to explain these terms to the patient. References are available to assist pharmacists in the wording to use for discussing some of these issues.[33]

It is also important for the pharmacist to be prepared to discuss apparent clinical changes that a patient may report after receiving a substituted brand medication. Although generic and brand-name drug products have the same active ingredients, some patients apparently experience slightly different effects from products manufactured by different manufacturers. These may be real or perceived effects.

When a patient reports such an effect, the pharmacist should treat it as any other report by a patient of an unexpected effect. The appropriate clinical aspects of the situation must be considered regarding the therapeutic outcome, as well as the patient's personal concerns.

In this situation, the pharmacist should focus on the patient's concerns and perceptions of the situation. The patient may be worried or afraid of the drug effects, as well as angry at the pharmacist, the physician, the government and/or the third-party payer.

The pharmacist should listen carefully to the patient and avoid making excuses or belittling the patient for perceiving problems that have been previously unreported. Every attempt should be made to calm the patient and validate his or her feelings. In this way, the situation is least likely to result in loss of confidence by the patient in the drug, the physician and the pharmacist.

Social (Preventative Health Care) Counseling

Although pharmacists deal with patients primarily in the area of medication counseling, they are also generally considered to be the most available health professionals in the community. It has been estimated that a number of people equivalent to the total population of the United States visits the more than 50,000 pharmacies in the country every 3 1/2 weeks.[34] The pharmacist may, therefore, be the first person that a patient will turn to in order to discuss a variety of problems. Not only is no appointment needed with the pharmacist, but the patient may feel more comfortable discussing personal matters with the pharmacist than with a more formal caregiver—especially if a helping and trusting relationship has developed between the patient and the pharmacist. Pharmacists are in a unique position, and therefore, have a responsibility to become involved in preventive health care.

Pharmacists' involvement in preventive health care includes primary and secondary prevention. Pharmacists become involved in secondary prevention through prescription and nonprescription counseling by detecting problems and optimizing therapy.[34] Involvement in primary prevention, however, requires pharmacists to promote health maintenance in individual patients by providing education on topics such as smoking, alcohol use, nutrition, exercise, etc.[34] Although pharmacists have not generally actively pursued this role, they often become involved when they are approached by patients to answer questions about drugs or illness and, in some cases, about social problems.

Drug-Related and Illness-Related Questions

Many pharmacies now provide a patient-information section in the pharmacy that holds pamphlets and patient-oriented reference books regarding not only medications, but also various illness conditions. Patients should be encouraged to discuss this information with the pharmacist at any time. In addition, pharmacists often become involved in national health observances such as National Mental Health Month, National Arthritis Month, etc., or hold store promotions related to a particular condition, thus inviting questions from the public. Pharmacists involved in screening for hypertension, diabetes, or colorectal cancer also need to be prepared to answer questions and discuss the condition with the patient.

In dealing with general questions about drugs or illness, it is best to gather some information about the request before responding. The pharmacist should find out why the patient wants to know, what specifically he wants to know, where he heard about the drug or illness in question, and what he already knows. This will allow the pharmacist to determine the nature of the patient's needs.

If a patient requests a reference book, it is preferable to provide prepared information pamphlets or books designed specifically for patients, such as those suggested in Appendix A. It is not advisable to simply hand the patient a pharmacists' reference text, which is too detailed and technical for most patients to understand and may indeed be mystifying, alarming, or misleading. If the patient is familiar with and requests to see a particular pharmacists' reference text, the pharmacist should not appear to be withholding information. In cases where it would be awkward to refuse to show the book to the patient, the pharmacist should stay with the patient and ask questions as suggested above, to determine the patient's needs or concerns. The pharmacist can then help to clarify the information in the reference in terms that the patient can more easily understand, and put the information into perspective.

Often the result of this type of discussion will be a suggestion that the patient make an appointment with his physician.

Nondrug-Related Concerns

Patients may also approach the pharmacist with nondrug-related concerns, or alternatively, the pharmacist may become aware of these concerns through discussion or observation. These concerns may include personal or family problems such as alcoholism, drug abuse, family planning, unwanted pregnancy, child abuse or family violence, and suicidal thoughts.

Patients may not know where to get help for their problems, or they may not be quite ready to seek more formal care. Patients in these situations need assistance finding out where they can get more specialized help for their problems. They may need confirmation that they indeed have a specific problem that can and should be treated. They may need encouragement to seek help. They may also need reassurance about the source of referred help regarding confidentiality and the nature of the encounter with that caregiver. Finally, they may need some help in the practical aspects of accessing or contacting that source.

Although we speak of "patient counseling," pharmacists are not trained to "counsel" in any but drug-related situations, while social counseling situations often require professional counselors. Since pharmacists are approached, however, they have a responsibility to deal with the patient rather than turning him or her away. Regarding child abuse, pharmacists are professionally, and in some states, legally responsible to report suspected cases to the proper authorities.[35]

Dealing with Patients' Nondrug-Related Concerns

1. *Listen.* The pharmacist should be prepared to listen in an unbiased and nonjudgmental manner. As with other counseling situations, the pharmacist should begin by allowing the patient to express his or her feelings or concerns, empathizing with the patient. Some gentle probing may be needed for the pharmacist to get a full understanding of the patient's needs.

2. *Encourage Patients to Seek Their Own Solutions.* The pharmacist should avoid giving advice, even if asked directly—instead, he should stress that such decisions are up to the patient. The pharmacist can help the patient to explore some options.

3. *Refer Patients to Appropriate Helpers.* In order to handle these situations properly, the pharmacist must be familiar with resources in the community to which the patient can be referred. Such sources include physicians; specialized clinics (e.g., family planning clinics); priests, ministers or rabbis; school counselors; specialized treatment centers (e.g., addiction treatment center); self-help organizations (e.g., Alcoholics Anonymous); crisis-intervention services (e.g., suicide hotlines); and social-service agencies.

    It is useful to keep a list of referral resources, with phone numbers and the name of a contact person, if available. When making up such a list, it may also be helpful for the pharmacist to contact the resources personally to find out about their referral procedures and the sort of treatment the patient can expect to receive from them. This way, the pharmacist will feel more confident in making referrals and may be able to reassure patients by explaining what will happen when they reach the particular helper.

4. *Follow-up.* The pharmacist might also engage in follow-up counseling to see if the patient was able to contact the referred resource, informing the patient in advance that he will do so. This will encourage and reassure the patient that the recommended help is indeed necessary and that he can rely on the support of a concerned individual.

5. *Provide Privacy.* Because these situations are of a very personal nature, the pharmacist should be sensitive to the need for privacy. If a private

area is not available for the discussion, a time might be arranged to speak with the patient when there will be privacy in the pharmacy. Alternatively, the pharmacist might arrange to speak with the patient on the telephone.

6. *Ensure Confidentiality.* The pharmacist should keep in mind the need to maintain confidentiality. If, in the pharmacist's opinion, someone else should be informed about the situation—a physician, parent, family member, or social-service worker —he or she must first discuss it with the patient. Patients should be encouraged to first speak with these people themselves. If a patient feels unable to do this, the pharmacist may offer to intervene, but only with the patient's consent. The only exception to this rule would be in the case of child abuse, as mentioned above, where the pharmacist is legally responsible for reporting any suspected incidents, and may not want to discuss it further with the patient.[35] In any of these cases, discussion of the patient's situation with other pharmacy staff or with acquaintances must also be restricted.

Throughout any discussion with the patient, confidentiality should be emphasized to encourage and comfort the patient.

Summary

A lot has been written in the previous chapters about what pharmacists *should* do regarding patient counseling, however the question arises as to how the average pharmacist in everyday practice *is able to* accomplish this. This chapter in particular highlights some of the difficulties for pharmacists with respect to performing this important duty. The following chapter will further discuss difficulties facing pharmacists in patient counseling and will offer some practical suggestions for pharmacists to overcome some of these difficulties and develop optimal counseling involvement.

References

1. Morrow N, Hargie O. An investigation of critical incidents in interpersonal communication in pharmacy practice. J Soc Admin Pharm. 1987;4(3): 112-118.
2. Klein L, German P, Levine D, et al. Medication problems among outpatients: A study with emphasis on the elderly. Arch Intern Med.1984;144 (6):1185-1188.
3. Schoepp G. For kids only. Drug Merch. 1990;71(1):26-31.
4. Mechanic D. Illness behavior. In. Medical Sociology. 2nd ed. New York: Free Press. 1978.
5. Eigen B. Improving communication with the physically disabled. Am Pharm. 1982;NS22(10):37-40.
6. Penna R. Pharmacists should make appointments to serve patients with chronic diseases. Am Pharm. 1991;NS31(7):57-59.
7. Work D. We've come a long way... or have we? Am Pharm. 1987;NS27(7): 48-50.

8. Weygman L. Managing conflict. On Cont Pract. 1988;15(1):19-20.
9. Myerscough P. Aspects of transcultural communication. In: Talking with patients—A basic clinical skill. 2nd Ed. Oxford: Oxford University Press. 1992.
10. Wilson J, Hogan L. Readability testing of auxiliary labels. Drug Intell Clin Pharm.1983;17(1):54-55.
11. Hurd P, Butkovich S. Compliance problems and the older patient: Assessing functional limitations. Drug Intell Clin Pharm. 1986;20(3):228-230.
12. Miller B. Break sound barrier with the deaf person in your pharmacy. Drug Merch. 1984;65(10):44.
13. Chermak G, Jinks M. Counseling the hearing-impaired older adult. Drug Intell Clin Pharm.1981;15(5):377-382.
14. Myerscough P. Other aspects of doctor-patient communication. In: Talking with patients—A basic clinical skill. 2nd Ed. Oxford: Oxford University Press. 1992.
15. Torre M, Sause R. Counseling the diabetic patient. Am Pharm. 1982;NS22(10):45-46.
16. Raleigh F. Counseling the patient with psychiatric conditions. Cal Pharm. 1990;Feb:33-35.
17. Okolo N, McReynolds J. Counseling the terminally ill. Am Pharm. 1987;NS27(9):37-40.
18. Buckman R. I don't know what to say. Toronto: Key Porter Books Ltd. 1988.
19. Billow J, Mort J, Vreugdenhil D, et al. Tips on communicating with the elderly. Am Pharm. 1991;NS31(4):51-54.
20. Currie CT. Talking to the elderly. In: Talking with patients—A basic clinical skill. 2nd Ed. Oxford: Oxford University Press. 1992.
21. Galizia V, Sause R. Communicating with the geriatric patient. Am Pharm. 1982;NS22(10):35-36.
22. Epstein D. What older patients want from you. Drug Topics.1991;135(5):50-52,55.
23. Culbertson V, Arthur T, Rhodes P, et al. Consumer preferences for verbal and written medication information. Drug Intell Clin Pharm. 1988;22(5):390-396.
24. Green L, Mullen P, Stainbrook G. Programs to reduce drug errors in the elderly: Direct and indirect evidence from patient education. J Ger Drug Ther. 1986;1(1):3-18.
25. Ascione F, Shimp L. the effectiveness of four educational strategies in the elderly. Drug Intell Clin Pharm. 1984;18(11):926-931.
26. Tett S, Higgins G, Armour C. Impact of pharmacist interventions on medication management by the elderly. A review of the literature. Am Pharmacother. 1993;27(1):80-86.
27. Covington T. Whitney Jr H. Patient-pharmacist communication techniques. Drug Intell Clin Pharm. 1971;5(11):370-376.

28. Gerrard BA, Boniface W, Love B. Developing skills for coping with interpersonal stress. In. Interpersonal Skills for Health Professionals. Reston, VA: Reston Publishing. 1980.
29. Steptoe A. Psychophysiological processes in disease. In Health Care and Human Behaviour. Steptoe A, Mathews A., eds. London: Academic Press. 1984.
30. Albro W. Dealing with difficult patients. Pharm Student. 1992;Feb:13-15.
31. Parker R, Martinez D, Covington T. Drug product selection-Part 1: History and legal overview. Am Pharm.1991;NS31(7):72-78.
32. Shargel L, Yu A. Bioavailability and bioequivalence. In. Applied Biopharmaceutics and Pharmacokinetics. 3rd ed. East Norwalk, CT: Appleton-Century-Crofts. 1993.
33. United States Pharmacopeial Convention, Inc. About the medicines you are taking. In. About Your Medicines. 6th ed. Rockville, MD:USPC, 1991.
34. Jinks M, Cornely P, Mayer F. The pharmacist's role in individual preventive health care. Am Pharm. 1983;NS23(7):10-17.
35. Mangione R. The pharmacist's role in child abuse prevention. Am J Pharm Ed.1988;52(3):161-163.

9
DEVELOPING OPTIMAL COUNSELING INVOLVEMENT

Thus far, this book has provided pharmacists with some theory and background information about patient counseling in order to provide an appropriate perspective for counseling. In addition, some practical aspects of counseling have been discussed concerning the content of counseling, materials and techniques, and skills required. Having read this, however, a pharmacy student may say: "We're taught in pharmacy school to counsel patients, but I don't see it happening in many pharmacies that I walk into. Why is that, and what can I do to make things different?" As the pharmacy student observed, many pharmacists find it difficult to become involved in patient counseling to the extent required today by professional and regulatory standards. This chapter will make suggestions to assist pharmacists in developing optimal counseling involvement.

Barriers to Effective Patient Counseling

Less than half of consumers report in surveys that they receive verbal information for new prescriptions, even fewer for refill prescriptions.[1,2,3] The majority of pharmacists report that they would like to spend more time counseling patients and that counseling is their most preferred activity.[4,5,6]

It appears that, although the majority of pharmacists want to be more involved in patient counseling, they are finding it difficult to provide this service. What, then, is preventing pharmacists from becoming more involved in patient counseling?

In one survey of practicing pharmacists, respondents offered more than 50 "excuses" for not communicating with patients.[7] Pharmacists are apparently confronted by many barriers to making patient counseling part of their regular activities.[7,8] Ten major barriers seem to present most of the problems (see Table 9.1). Some of these barriers involve practical issues such as lack of time, economic considerations, and physical barriers. Other barriers are presented by patients—either through their lack of awareness of the need for counseling and its availability, through their perceptions of the pharmacist as simply a drug dispenser, or through comprehension difficulties. In addition, pharmacists may personally create barriers through lack of confidence, knowledge, or communication skills, and through their poor relationship with physicians.

Practical Barriers to Patient Counseling

The most commonly cited factor preventing pharmacists from becoming involved in patient counseling is lack of time.[7,8] Pharmacists report that the greatest source of stress in their jobs is lack of time (being interrupted, not having enough staff to provide necessary services, having so much work that everything cannot be done well).[9] Part of the difficulty seems to be the type of activities that pharmacists engage in. Pharmacists report that 30% of their time is spent in non-pharmaceutical activities, and acknowledge that this is too much.[5]

Table 9.1   Barriers to Patient Counseling

Lack of time

Physical barriers (lack of privacy; inaccessibility of the pharmacist)

Economic considerations

Patient's poor perception of the pharmacist

Lack of awareness on the part of the patient of the need for counseling and of

    its availability

Comprehension difficulties

Lack of knowledge (about drugs and the patient's history)

Lack of confidence

Poor physician–pharmacist relationship

Poor communication skills

Adapted from Gossel TA. A pharmacist's perspective on improving patient communication. Guidelines to Professional Pharmacy. 1980;7(3):1,4,5; Knapp DA. Barriers faced by pharmacists when attempting to maximaze their contribution to society. Am J Pharm Educ. 1979;43(4):357-359.

The traditional layout of pharmacies presents a physical barrier to pharmacists' patient-counseling activities.[7,8] Traditionally, pharmacists have been confined to the dispensing area of the pharmacy. In hospital pharmacies, this area is often far removed from the usual flow of patients, sometimes with only a small wicket for access to the pharmacist. Community pharmacies often have the floor level of the dispensing area raised above the rest of the pharmacy, with high barriers and counters often obscuring the patient's view of the pharmacist. Such physical barriers have been shown to create a negative attitude in the patient toward the pharmacist.[10] They make it difficult for the pharmacist to interact with the patient, and inhibit discussion of personal information. Many pharmacies afford little or no opportunity for private discussion between the patient and the pharmacist. Most patients report that they want privacy, preferably in the form of a private consulting area in the pharmacy.[2,11]

Other physical factors, such as the decor of the area—the use of color and the arrangement of furnishings—as well as lighting and noise levels, may also affect patient–pharmacist communication.[12]

Finally, economic considerations present a practical barrier to patient counseling.[7,8] Since patient counseling requires time, it can result in the need for extra staff, thereby increasing the pharmacy department's overhead. In fact, estimates indicate that the cost of counseling may be $1 to $2 per prescription (not including the cost of establishing a patient profile or interventions where the pharmacist must take action such as telephoning the physician).[12] Some pharmacists are unwilling to provide counseling services until patients or third-party providers pay for them.

Patients Barriers to Counseling

Although pharmacists may be willing to counsel patients, they often perceive patients to be unwilling to ask their advice about nonprescription medications or to participate in patient counseling about prescriptions.[7,8]

The results of many studies of the public's perception of pharmacists belie the notion that such barriers exist, since most patients report that they do in fact want information from their pharmacist.[1,2,3]

A more realistic barrier to patient counseling is the variety of comprehension difficulties that face pharmacists during patient counseling.[7,8] As discussed in the previous chapter, comprehension difficulties may include not only the patient's difficulties in speaking the English language because of foreign origin, but also difficulties in comprehension owing to the patient's low literacy level. The pharmacist's technical jargon and various patients' disabilities can also inhibit patient comprehension.

Pharmacist Barriers to Patient Counseling

Pharmacists are sometimes reluctant to become involved in patient counseling because of a lack of confidence in their abilities in patient counseling and in their pharmaceutical knowledge.[7,8]

Some pharmacists fear that the patient will ask a question that they cannot answer. They are often unsure of their knowledge base and worry about not being able to provide all the information that might be required. In these times, because new drugs are continually being developed, it can be difficult for the pharmacist to keep abreast of current information.

Pharmacists are generally required to complete mandatory continuing education (C.E.), but it may be necessary for pharmacists to do more than the minimum required, particularly for speciality areas of practice.

Lack of knowledge about the patient's medical and medication history may also be a barrier to counseling.[7,8] Pharmacists can generally gather much of the information they need directly from the patient, provided that they ask in an appropriate manner. However, additional information may be needed from the physician or from hospital records.

That leads to another barrier to patient counseling, the pharmacist–physician relationship.[7,8] Some pharmacists believe that physicians do not appreciate pharmacists' involvement with their patients, and may in fact consider it an infringement on their territory. As discussed in Chapter 7, physician–pharmacist relationships need to be developed and nurtured for pharmacists to fulfil their roles in pharmaceutical care. Studies of the pharmacist–physician relationship indicate that physicians are cautious about certain pharmacist activities, such as recommending nonprescription products.[14,15]

Studies indicate that, although there are areas of tension between physicians and pharmacists, physicians are generally willing to work together with pharmacists for the benefit of the patient, rather than quarrelling with them over professional "turf."[14,15]

Another barrier that pharmacists themselves present to patient counseling is their own lack of communication skills when interacting with physicians and with patients.[14,15] The importance of communication skills for pharmacists was discussed at length in the previous chapter, and problems of pharmacists in this area have been identified.[16,17]

If pharmacists could improve their ability to communicate, they would not only be able to overcome their lack of confidence in this area, but would also be encouraged to remove other barriers to patient counseling by, for example, making the time for it and eliminating existing physical barriers.[18]

Removing the Barriers: The Four A's for Effective and Efficient Patient Counseling

The barriers to counseling may vary for each pharmacist and with each practice setting. Pharmacists must therefore analyze their own situations to see where barriers exist and how they may be overcome. To assist them in this analysis, pharmacists can consider the requirements for effective and efficient counseling and evaluate which requirements exist, and which need to be improved.

The requirements for conducting a counseling session in an effective and efficient manner can be summarized in four words: *availability, atmosphere, attitude,* and *approach.*

Availability

First of all, pharmacists must make themselves available to patients. The patient must know who the pharmacist is and be able to interact with him or her easily.

To increase the pharmacist's availability to the patient, attempts must be made to remove the many physical barriers in the pharmacy.[18] The pharmacist must be visible in order for patients to see that there is a pharmacist on duty. A low prescription counter without barriers of plexiglass or stacked products along the divider will allow the patient to see the pharmacist and show that he or she is available.

In addition, the pharmacist should be identifiable and in some way distinct from the other pharmacy staff, by wearing a name tag and a distinctive lab coat or uniform.

The pharmacy layout must also be evaluated to assure that it allows for easy access by the pharmacist to the counseling areas, as well as to the nonprescription drug area.[12,13,19] Although many pharmacies are now providing private counseling areas, these are often at a distance from the dispensing area, and are therefore inconvenient for the pharmacist to use.[20] Figure 9.1 shows some suggested pharmacy layouts to allow maximum availability of the pharmacist.

The pharmacy layout behind the prescription counter must also be evaluated to determine how well it provides a work flow that allows the pharmacist to be available to patients. Pharmacists need assistance with the dispensing function in order to allow them to interact more with patients. Different states have different regulations regarding what pharmacy technicians (also termed "ancillary," "supportive," or "nonlicensed" personnel) can do, if indeed they are recognized at all.[21] Where allowed by regulation, the pharmacy technician should perform the necessary technical tasks, allowing the pharmacist the freedom to talk to patients. Ideally, the pharmacist should receive the prescription, so that he or she can check any initial details with the patient, and arrange to conduct a medication-history interview if necessary. The pharmacy technician should prepare the prescription, entering the necessary information into the computer. The pharmacist should then check the patient's medication profile, and check the prescription, then proceed to counsel the patient.

Although the pharmacy technician should perform the bulk of computer functions, the pharmacist will also need access to the computer records to review the patient's medication history before checking the prescription and while counseling the patient. If two computer screens are not available, the patient's most recent drug history could be printed out with the prescription label, allowing the pharmacist to review it when checking the prescription and refer to it when talking to the patient. In addition, computer programs are now available to assist in identifying problems such as adverse drug reactions, duplication, interactions, allergies, etc.[22] As a result, the pharmacy technician should be able to perform most of the computer functions, alerting the pharmacist when problems are indicated through the computer program.

Although pharmacy technicians play an essential role in the pharmacy, neither they nor store clerks should act as intermediaries between the patient and the pharmacist. The pharmacist should be free to interact personally with the patient and should be the only person who counsels the patient.

Even if the pharmacist is physically available for consultation, the patient may not perceive him or her to be available. The reason patients often give for not talking to their pharmacist is that they think he or she is too busy. The pharmacist must make the time to talk with the patient. This means that the time allotted to fill each prescription must include an allowance for time spent interacting with the patient.

Figure 9.1 Suggested Pharmacy Layouts for Effective and Efficient Patient Counseling

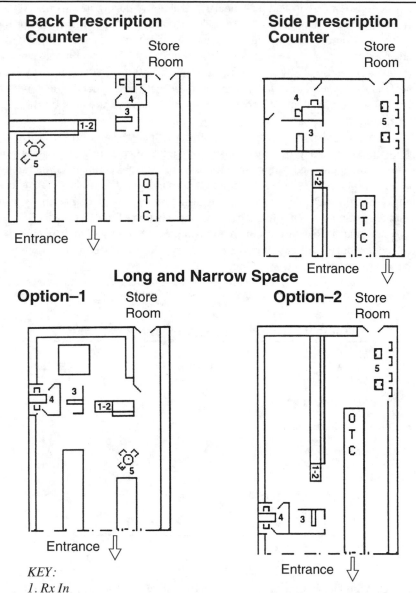

Back Prescription Counter
Store Room

Entrance

Side Prescription Counter
Store Room

Entrance

Long and Narrow Space

Option–1
Store Room

Entrance

Option–2
Store Room

Entrance

KEY:
1. Rx In
2. Cash Register
3. Semiprivate counseling area
4. Private counseling area
5. Waiting area and information center

Note: These drawings are not to scale and may need to be adapted to meet regulatory standards

In order for a pharmacist to be available to each patient, it may in some cases be necessary to increase pharmacy staff, with either additional pharmacy technicians or an additional pharmacist, particularly during peak times. If the situation demands a longer and more in-depth discussion than is practical during the normal flow of work, arrangements can be made with the patient to talk with the pharmacist later on the telephone. The pharmacist can further manage his or her time for counseling by scheduling appointments either in the pharmacy or at the patient's home, at a mutually convenient time.[23] These special arrangements will allow the pharmacist to conduct longer counseling sessions during less hectic times in the pharmacy.

To further demonstrate their availability for patient counseling to patients, pharmacists should promote themselves in the community as sources of information about medications and illness. Advertising campaigns, including posters, in-pharmacy signs, and pamphlets can increase the public's awareness in this regard.[21-26] Displays of patient-information leaflets in the pharmacy also heighten awareness that information provision is part of the pharmacist's role.

Pharmacists can further enhance the public's awareness of their availability by reaching out to their communities through speaking to community groups and schools as discussed in Chapter 6.[27]

A summary of the methods for pharmacists to improve their availability for counseling is shown in Table 9.2.

Table 9.2 Improving Pharmacist Availability

Visibility of the pharmacist

Organization of the pharmacy

Use of technicians

Computer arrangements

Access to counseling areas

Managing time

Making appointments

Promotion of pharmacist's role and community activities

Atmosphere

Even if the pharmacist is available, the patient may not be prepared to talk particularly about personal matters. Sometimes pharmacists forget that the nature of a patient's illness and medication use is very personal. An atmosphere is needed in which a patient can feel comfortable asking the pharmacist's advice and discussing his or her prescription and illness. Consumers report in surveys that they would prefer a private consulting area in the pharmacy.[2,11]

Although it is often difficult to arrange for a completely private counseling area, a more private atmosphere can be created in a number of ways. Reducing physical barriers and removing the raised platform of the dispensary, or at least providing a step down at the counter can allow the pharmacist to get physically closer to the patient, lessening the feeling of intimidation for the patient, and increasing the feeling of intimacy. The pharmacist might also lead the patient away from the counter, possibly into a quieter aisle, and position herself so that the patient is between her and the wall, thus creating a private corner.

An atmosphere of privacy can also be achieved through the use of a semi-private counseling area. Signs or partial dividers can be used to indicate to other waiting patients that an area is designated for private counseling, discouraging them from crowding the patient being counseled. A waiting area that is out of earshot of the counseling area can also help to create a greater degree of privacy.

For effective and efficient patient counseling, the pharmacy layout should ideally provide a number of counseling areas, including a semiprivate and a private area (see Figure 9.1). The majority of the counseling sessions could be carried out in the semi-private area, close to the prescription counter. Situations that require more privacy, such as those that involve an embarrassed or upset patient or that call for a more detailed discussion, can be conducted in the private area. The private counseling area could also be used for pre-arranged appointments with patients for further in-depth discussions of their medications.

Many pharmacies are now being designed to remove physical barriers and provide more privacy for counseling. Some examples of private and semiprivate counseling areas and of a waiting area are shown in Figures 9.2, 9.3, and 9.4.

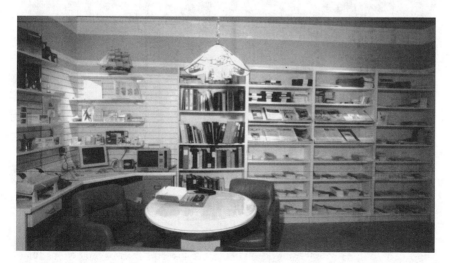

Figure 9.2 *Private counseling room at Brant Arts Pharmacy, Burlington, Ontario, Canada.*

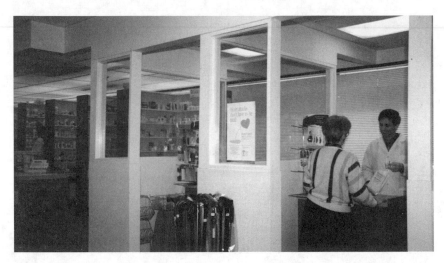

Figure 9.3 Semiprivate counseling booth at King Medical Arts Pharmacy and Home Health Care in Mississauga, Ontario, Canada.

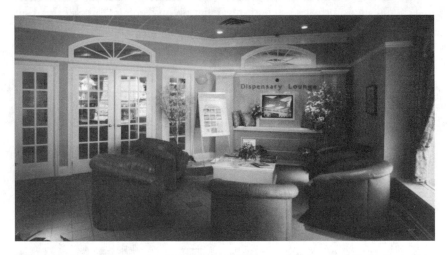

Figure 9.4 Waiting area at Brant Arts Pharmacy, Burlington, Ontario, Canada.

The pharmacist can also enhance the atmosphere of intimacy through the use of nonverbal language.[10] To create the sense of a personal conversation rather than of a lecture, the pharmacist should position himself or herself within 2 to 4 feet of the patient. Using a quieter tone of voice, maintaining eye contact, and slightly inclining the body forward will help create a more personal and intimate atmosphere.

The general atmosphere of the pharmacy can also contribute to effective counseling. By removing clutter from the counter area and reducing noise levels (such as loud music or loud telephone bells), the pharmacist can make the environment even more conducive to conversation.[12,28] Some background music however, is desirable, since it reduces the ability of waiting patients to overhear the pharmacist's conversations with other patients.

Ways that pharmacists can improve the pharmacy atmosphere are summarized in Table 9.3.

Table 9.3   Improving Pharmacy Atmosphere

Provide a private counseling area

Provide a semiprivate counseling area

Use nonverbal language to create a sense of personal conversation

Improve the general atmosphere

Approach

The third requirement for effective counseling involves the pharmacist's approach to each individual counseling situation. In order to be effective and efficient, the pharmacist should have a systematic and organized approach to any situation that a patient presents, at all times taking into consideration the specific patient and the specific situation.

Since the pharmacist has quite a lot to think about when counseling a patient (in addition to medication information), it will help to have a specific plan, or protocol, to follow. Following an organized protocol, as suggested in Chapter 5, will allow the pharmacist to grasp the situation and identify the facts involved quickly. Having an idea of specific words, actions, and sequences to use can take some of the guesswork out of counseling, allowing the pharmacist to cover the necessary information in a minimum amount of time. See Appendix B for suggested dialogues for counseling.

Another element of an efficient and effective approach is tailoring counseling to the particular patient and situation. As described in Chapter 8, by considering the specific characteristics of the patient, the drug, and the situation, the pharmacist can focus his or her time on the areas most critical to effective medication use by the patient.

The most important aspect of the pharmacist's approach to patient counseling involves the helping model approach discussed in Chapter 2. This approach places the focus of counseling on the patient, allowing him to participate in his own treatment and to decide for himself what he needs to know and what problems he needs to overcome for his therapy to be most effective. It also allows the pharmacist to focus on the most important areas for that particular patient.

The pharmacist must also develop good communication skills, as discussed in Chapter 7, if he or she is to apply the helping approach effectively. The pharmacist needs to establish conditions for effective communication, in particular, a helping relationship. The pharmacist must employ communication skills such as listening skills, to encourage the patient to identify his or her counseling needs and concerns. Above all, the pharmacist must allow the counseling session to be a two-way communication process, and interviewing skills will assist in doing this.

The pharmacist can further improve the efficiency and effectiveness of counseling by employing the appropriate educational approach as discussed in Chapter 6. The pharmacist should take into consideration adult educational principles and various factors such as the goals of the counseling session when selecting the specific educational methods for the patient. In addition, pharmacists should use an appropriate selection of the many counseling aids available or develop ones to suit the individual patient's needs. These techniques to improve the pharmacist's approach to counseling are summarized in Table 9.4.

Table 9.4   Improving the Pharmacist's Approach to Counseling

Use an organized approach and protocol

Tailor counseling

Adopt a helping approach

Develop good communication skills

Use appropriate educational methods and counseling aids

Attitude

The pharmacist's attitude toward counseling itself and toward individual patients will contribute further towards effective and efficient counseling.

The pharmacist should maintain a professional but relaxed attitude, ensuring that he or she does not appear to be in a rush. Awareness of nonverbal language is important.[29] In the course of gathering information, an attentive attitude and posture that conveys interest and concern will be most likely to encourage the patient to talk.

If patients are to be willing to spend the time necessary for counseling with the pharmacist, they must be convinced that it is to their benefit. As discussed in Chapter 7, by maintaining an assertive attitude during the session, the pharmacist will indicate to the patient that it is important to listen and to understand.

The pharmacist should try to persuade patients that taking their medication is in their best interest, rather than to simply give orders to patients. As discussed in Chapter 4, the pharmacist should realize that it must be the patient's decision to follow a recommended course of therapy.

Pharmacists should also try to develop an attitude of confidence in their knowledge. Although they certainly *must* keep abreast of current pharmacology and therapeutics, they should also realize that, in most cases, they already possess a vast store of information that is likely to be sufficient for most counseling situations. Most questions from patients are fairly simple, and the majority of patients require quite basic information. Where more complex information is required, it is quite appropriate for the pharmacist to defer the answer to a later time, and consult a reference text or a drug-information center. It is important, of course, to arrange with the patient how and when the answer will be provided and to make a point of following through.

Pharmacists can become more confident in their knowledge by attending the many available continuing education programs, reading journals, taking correspondence courses, etc. In addition, computer software is becoming more and more available to assist the pharmacist in reviewing patient profiles to assess risk and identify problems.

New developments in information storage and retrieval are also making it easier for pharmacists to access patient's medical data, allowing pharmacists to be more confident discussing patients' therapies with physicians. Computer networking and technologies such as "smart cards" will further allow patients' medication information to be shared between pharmacies and physicians and amongst pharmacies.[30]

Finally, the pharmacist's attitude toward counseling itself is most important to becoming an efficient and effective patient counselor. The pharmacist must be convinced that being involved in patient counseling is vitally important for the profession, for the image of his or her practice or hospital department, and for personal satisfaction.

For some pharmacists, this conviction requires the assurance that they will be remunerated for patient-counseling services. Payment for these services does in fact occur in some pharmacy practices today, and patients have shown willingness to pay for counseling in the pharmacy and for private home consultation.[32,33,34]

Some pharmaceutical and insurance companies have also begun to reimburse pharmacists for patient counseling in specific instances such as diabetic counseling and medication reviews.

Even without direct payments, pharmacists' efforts to improve patient compliance through patient counseling can be not only cost-effective, but also financially rewarding, because they tend to result in increased refill prescriptions and in general a strengthening of customer loyalty.[35,36]

Ways that pharmacists can improve their attitudes to patient counseling are summarized in Table 9.5.

Table 9.5   Improving the Pharmacist's Attitude

Attend to nonverbal messages

Be assertive

Be persuasive

Be confident

Be a life-long learner

Take advantage of new technologies

Be a believer

Self-Development of the Counseling Pharmacist

The major barriers to patient counseling, as well as ways for pharmacists to analyze their own practices to maximize efficiency and effectiveness of counseling, have now been discussed.

For pharmacists who are just starting to counsel patients or who still feel that counseling is an overwhelming task, there are a series of steps that may help them develop into "counseling pharmacists." These steps are summarized in Table 9.6.

Table 9.6   Self Development of the Counseling Pharmacist

Assess your own values and priorities

Evaluate barriers

Arrange for removal or reduction of barriers where possible

Obtain counseling aids

Prepare staff, physicians, and patients

Prepare for each counseling session

Progress into counseling step-by-step

Remember to be assertive and to tailor counseling

Arrange for practice

Conduct a self-evaluation

Assessing Values and Priorities

Becoming involved in patient counseling may mean a change in the pharmacy's physical layout, a reorganization of time, and an investment in personal development for the pharmacist and others. Because this can require an expenditure of time and money, involving some major changes for the pharmacist, pharmacists must be convinced that counseling is important and worthwhile, and must be committed to the concept.

Pharmacists should review the benefits that counseling can bring to them and to their patients as discussed in Chapter 1. If these benefits correspond to the pharmacist's values, he or she will be prepared to embark on the necessary personal and professional development.

On a more practical level, pharmacists should also consider their professional duties and rank them in order of priority within their professional role, from "immediate" to "mid-range," "low," and "complete waste of time."[37]

Immediate: Duties that the pharmacist considers critical to his or her role or to the health of the patient. (The pharmacist committed to patient counseling would consider patient counseling an immediate priority.)

Mid-Range: Duties that are important to the role of the pharmacist, but have a lesser urgency in terms of time—they can more easily be rescheduled or reorganized (e.g., calling physicians, checking prescriptions).

Low Priority: Routine duties necessary for the operation of the prescription department and, possibly, of the whole pharmacy or the pharmacy department. They include placing orders, seeing sales representatives, doing administrative paperwork, and organizing staffing.

Although these functions are critical to the day-to-day running of the pharmacy, they are to a certain degree amenable to scheduling at the pharmacist's convenience. Some of them need not be performed by the pharmacist alone, and staff retraining might allow them to be undertaken, in full or in part, by nonpharmacist staff. For example, a nonprofessional staff member might be assigned to meet with sales representatives, with the pharmacist making the final approval of purchase orders.

Complete Waste of Time: Interruptions during a day that pharmacists endure, sometimes out of politeness, other times out of a lack of control. The pharmacist should consider such things as telephone calls that are unrelated to pharmacy, inventory functions (stocking, unpacking, ordering), answering the delivery door, and day-to-day staffing functions as unnecessary interruptions. Through a combination of delegation and reorganization, the pharmacist can minimize such interruptions in his or her working day.

Evaluating Barriers to Patient Counseling

As discussed in the previous section, there are many barriers to patient counseling. These vary with the practice situation and with the pharmacist. Pharmacists must evaluate their work environment and themselves to determine the barriers that are operative for them.

This requires an honest and in-depth evaluation. If barriers are overlooked at this point, attempts at patient counseling are destined to become frustrating.

Arranging for Removal or Reduction of Barriers

In the previous section, some suggestions were made for the removal or reduction of some of the barriers to patient counseling. Some barriers such as lack of confidence, poor communication skills, or lack of knowledge can be overcome through extra continuing-education activities, particularly workshops. Keeping up with new information can also be assisted by subscribing to journals and by joining a professional journal club.

Overcoming other barriers—for example, reorganizing the physical layout of the pharmacy—may be costly or require significant amounts of time. There may, however, be some financial assistance available through tax credits for modification that would accommodate disabled persons.[20]

Any major changes undertaken to remove barriers to counseling must be made with full consideration of their effects on the pharmacy's staff. Staff members should be made aware of the purpose of the changes, and even be made party to some of the planning. A front store clerk with many years of experience, for example, may become accustomed to answering questions about nonprescription medications. When the pharmacist resolves to become more involved in nonprescription counseling, he or she must make it a priority to explain to the clerk that this role is now to fall exclusively within the domain of the pharmacist's duties. This situation requires tact and assertiveness and, if ignored or mishandled, can lead to disgruntled staff and confused patients.

Obtaining Counseling Aids

As discussed previously in Chapter 6, there are a variety of counseling aids that can be used to assist the pharmacist. Appendix A includes a list of sources for patient information. A form letter can be composed and sent to each source, ordering patient-information leaflets. As discussed in Chapter 6, the pharmacist should evaluate all such materials for readability and appropriateness, and should be familiar with their contents.

The pharmacist should also arrange for the convenient storage of counseling aids, so that they are available at the time of counseling. In addition, a display area may be provided in the waiting area for patient-information materials, and possibly a video-tape machine may be made available.

Preparing Staff, Physicians, and Patients

As mentioned above, pharmacy staff should be involved as much as possible in any reorganization relating to patient counseling. In addition, they should be trained appropriately to deal with any new duties they might acquire.

If other pharmacists are involved, they should be encouraged in their commitment to patient counseling, and arrangements should be made for appropriate training in counseling skills as required.

Nonpharmacist staff should be told how to respond to patients when asked about patient-counseling activities, new pharmacy layout, or staffing changes. They may also be given a procedure for introducing patients to the pharmacist when medication or health-related questions are mistakenly directed to them rather than to the pharmacist.

As discussed earlier, physicians may feel threatened by pharmacists providing information to their patients. To avoid problems in this area, it may be useful for the pharmacist to contact the physicians whose patients are regular clients of the pharmacy. The nature and purpose of the new patient-counseling service can be explained, and samples of any patient-education material supplied to patients can also be provided for the physician's perusal. The pharmacist should be careful to present this as a service the pharmacist is providing to complement the physician's efforts in this area, and for the ultimate benefit of the patient.

Patients, too, may wonder about the changes associated with a new patient-counseling service, such as a new pharmacy layout and staffing changes. They may also be wary of the pharmacist's increased interest in them. As discussed in Chapter 5, the counseling protocol should always include an explanation of the pharmacist's purpose in the counseling, in order to prepare the patient for the potentially personal nature of the discussion, as well as to get the patient's agreement to continue. It may also be advisable to send a form letter to the pharmacy's regular clientele to introduce the new service. This would not only prepare patients for the change in the nature of their interaction with the pharmacist, but promote the pharmacy and its services as well.

Preparing for Each Counseling Session

Before meeting with individual patients, the pharmacist should take a moment to prepare himself for the encounter in the following ways:

1. *Review Patient Record.* For a new patient, conduct a medication-history interview then review it for any problems that need to be discussed. For a returning patient, review the patient record for any problems.
2. *Organize.* Organize in your mind all the information that you must provide to the patient. If necessary, consult reference sources (see Appendix A).
3. *Select Materials.* Select any patient-counseling aids and educational materials to be used in the counseling session.
4. *Have the Medication Available.* If the prescription was prepared at an earlier time, instruct pharmacy technicians to leave the bag unsealed, allowing the pharmacist and the patient to look at the medication bottles at the time of counseling.
5. *Remember the Counseling Protocol.* Have the appropriate counseling protocol in mind (see Chapter 5).
6. *Have Patient Information Available.* During counseling, the pharmacist should have access to the patient's information in the form of a computer printout of the patient record or immediate access to the patient record via a computer terminal.

Progressing into Counseling Step by Step

Becoming a counseling pharmacist does not have to happen overnight. A pharmacist can progress into counseling step by step, as follows:

1. *Personally Interact with Each Patient.* To become accustomed to interacting with patients, the pharmacist can make a point of personally taking prescription orders from patients and giving out the completed prescriptions. This way, the pharmacist can simply introduce herself or himself to patients and go over the label directions with them, answering any questions that might arise.

2. *Provide Complete Counseling in Steps.* Once the pharmacist is comfortable speaking to patients in this manner, the pharmacist can embark on complete counseling sessions for one drug class only—say, antibiotics. To prepare for this, he or she can review the relevant pharmacology and therapeutics to provide appropriate information about the drugs in that class. The pharmacist can also practice expressing such information in language that most patients would comprehend and following the protocols suggested in Chapter 5.

   Once the pharmacist is comfortable with counseling for one class of drugs, he or she can gradually add other classes, until he or she feels confident conducting counseling sessions relating to all the drug classes.

3. *Provide Community Outreach.* The pharmacist may want to develop his or her communication skills further by giving presentations to community groups about the safe use of medications or by taking part in clinics, such as "brown-bag clinics" for the elderly, in which patients' drug use is reviewed.

Remembering to be Assertive and to Tailor Counseling

When developing counseling skills, pharmacists must remember that counseling should be tailored to individual patients and individual situations, as discussed in Chapter 8. They must consider where to place the emphasis in each counseling session and learn to make effective use of the information-gathering phase of the protocol to determine what is and what is not needed in each particular session.

Pharmacists who are anxious to provide patient-counseling services should be careful to avoid aggressiveness in their approach to counseling. They should remember that, in some situations, particularly those in which the patient is angry or upset, it may be counter-productive to proceed with the session at that time.

Practicing

For some pharmacists, it may be useful to practice patient counseling in order to feel more comfortable interacting with patients. One way to do this is to practice the dialogues suggested in Appendix B, using an audiotape or videotape recorder or simply by practicing in front of a mirror. Practice can help the pharmacist learn the order of the protocol and the suggested wordings of, say, the introduction or the discussion of side effects.

Another form of practice that may be helpful is role-playing, where participants assume an identity other than their own and are asked to cope with hypothetical problems. Mistakes can be made and observed, and alternative responses can be tried, allowing for experimentation in relatively nonthreatening circumstances with different ways of handling a situation.[38]

Role-playing should ideally be carried out with at least two players and one observer. Roles may include pharmacist and patient, nurse, physician, pharmacy technician, supervisor, and so on. Educational programs are available that use role-playing practice, and some of these are listed in Appendix A.

Self-Evaluation

Patient-counseling and communication skills can not be learned overnight or acquired through studying or reading a book. The pharmacist who resolves to become involved in patient counseling is embarking on a gradual process of learning and self-development. Each new counseling experience will build on the previous one. And, even after many years of patient counseling, pharmacists will be faced with new situations that may require new approaches.

To learn from and to evolve through these experiences, pharmacists should evaluate their performances after each counseling situation, taking the following elements into consideration:

1. The overall handling of the situation: Did the encounter end satisfactorily from the pharmacist's and patient's perspectives?
2. Was the goal of counseling accomplished? In other words, will it help the patient get the most benefit from his or her medication?
3. Was the pharmacist able to explain all the necessary information adequately, in terms that the patient could understand clearly?
4. Were the patient's concerns or problems resolved or, alternatively, were arrangements made to deal with them later?

The only way to evaluate some of these aspects of counseling is of course through follow-up counseling.

Pharmacists can also use videotape recordings to evaluate their tone of voice and nonverbal language, either in simulated, role-playing situations (as described above) or in real situations (with the permission of the patient). In their self-evaluations, pharmacists should make a point of identifying positive elements first, then should focus on the weaker aspects of their performance. They should keep in mind that there are no perfect counselors— not only because every patient is different, but because all pharmacists will, from time to time, find that hasty judgment calls are inescapable. There are simply degrees of comfort and satisfaction in counseling, and individual pharmacists can only strive to find the approaches and attitudes that make the exercise most productive, and most rewarding, for them and for their patients.

Summary

Understanding what counseling involves and the techniques to use is only half the battle. Pharmacists must find their own ways, in their individual practice situations, to arrange for patient counseling. This may mean some remodelling of the pharmacy, some extra staffing, and some extra reading and studying.

The critical element is the pharmacist's willingness to work at expanding patient-counseling activities and skills at his or her own pace. The profession of pharmacy has been evolving over hundreds of years, and each pharmacist can evolve, too, into an effective and efficient patient counselor. This evolution does not have to happen overnight, but regulatory and professional developments make change more urgent now than ever before.

References

1. Gannon K. Do you pass? Drug Topics. 1990:134(6):32-40.
2. Anon. Schering Report XIV. Kentucky Pharmacist. 1992: June:176-178.
3. Laverty R. Patients loyal but need the Rx information. Drug Topics. 1984:(5):38-40, 42-45.
4. Meade V. APhA survey looks at patient counseling. Am Pharm. 1992;NS32(4):27-29.
5. Chi J. How pharmacists feel about: Careers and workplace. Drug Topics. 1992;136(3):47,51,52,57.
6. Anon. Survey shows Rxers like counseling best. Drug Store News. 1986; Oct:48.
7. Gossel TA. A pharmacist's perspective on improving patient communication. Guidelines to Professional Pharmacy. 1980:7(3):1, 4, 5.
8. Knapp DA. Barriers faced by pharmacists when attempting to maximize their contribution to society. Am J Pharm Educ. 1979:43(4):357-359.
9. Ortmeier B, Wolfgang A. Jog-related stress: Perceptions of employee pharmacists. Am Pharm. 1991;NS31(9):27-31.
10. Ranelli PL. The utility of nonverbal communication in the profession of pharmacy. Soc Sci Med. 1979;13A(6): 1733-36.
11. Anon. NACDS study rates the value of some pharmacy services. Am Pharm.1992;NS32(4):5.
12. Polanski R, Polanski V. Environment for communication. Am Pharm. 1982; 22(10):545-546.
13. Anon. Perspectives in pharmacy economics. NACDS: The PipeLine. 1992;4(4):1.
14. Anon. 1984 Schering report explores pharmacist-physician relationship. Am Pharm. 1984;24(10):13-14.
15. Ortiz M, Thomas R. Attitudes of medical practitioners to community pharmacists giving medication advice to patients: Findings of a pharmacy practice foundation survey (Part 3). Australian J of Pharm. 1985;66(10): 803-810.

16. Baldwin J, McCroskey J, Knutson T. Communication apprehension in the pharmacy student. Am J Pharm Ed.1979;43(2):91-93.
17. Baldwin J, Richmond V, McCroskey J, et al. The quiet pharmacist. Am Pharm. 1982;NS22(10):536-539.
18. Baker E. Overcoming the barriers that prevent community pharmacists from maximizing their contributions to health care. Am J Pharm Ed. 1979;43(4):359-361.
19. Heard B. The pharmacy setting in patient counseling. On Cont Pract.1985;12(3):17-21.
20. Feegel K, Dix Smith M. Counseling and cognitive services for Medicaid patients under OBRA-90. Pharm Times.1992;9 Supp:1-9.
21. Ball S. Technicians: Boon or bane to busy pharmacists? Drug Store News. 1991:1(8):23, 24, 26, 28.
22. Cataldo R. Obra'90 and your pharmacy computer system. Am Pharm. 1992;NS32(11):39-41.
23. Penna R. Pharmacists should make appointments to serve patients with chronic diseases. Am Pharm. 1991;NS31(7):57-59.
24. Anon. Schering's "Ask Your Pharmacist" public service program underway. Am Druggist. 1984;189(3):94.
25. Anon. NCPIE'S Get the answers reaching millions of Americans. Am Pharm.1984;NS24(9):11-12.
26. Rantucci M, Segal H. Public awareness: An assessment of the public response to a display illustrating community pharmacists' roles and services. Can Pharm J.1984;117(6):272-275.
27. Nelson M. Our guest for tonight is...Pharmacists and public speaking. Am Pharm.1993;NS33(3):59-62.
28. Lively B. Communication as a transactional process: Basic tools of the community pharmacist. Contemp Pharm Pract.1978;1(2):81-85.
29. Samuelson K. Nonverbal messages can speak louder than words. Health Care.1986;Apr:12-13.
30. Jones J. Assessing potential risk of drugs: The elusive target. Ann Intern Med.1992;117(80):691-692.
31. Ritchey FJ, Raney MR. Effect of exposure on physicians' attitudes toward clinical pharmacists. Am J Hosp Pharm. 1981;38:1459-1463.
32. Anon. Customers at Wisconsin pharmacy pay for RPh's counseling services. Am Drug.1984;189(6):100.
33. Carroll N. Consumer demand for patient oriented services in community pharmacies—A review and comment. J Soc Admin Pharm.1985;3(2): 64-69.
34. Laverty R. Payment for services? Don't hold your breath. Drug Topics. 1984;128(6):18,19.
35. Jackson R, Huffman D. Patient compliance: The financial impact on your practice. NARD J. 1990;112(7):67-71.

36. Murphy D. Promoting compliance pays off. Am Pharm. 1985;25(1):19, 22, 23.
37. Weygman L. Time management. On Cont Pract.1988:15(3):27-28.
38. Beardsley W, Knapp D. Developing role-playing scenarios. Am J Pharm Educ. 1980;44(2):162-167.

APPENDIX A

RESOURCES
FOR PATIENT COUNSELING

Resources for Pharmacists to Use

Resources for Medication Information

Printed Resources

AHFS Drug Information. Bethesda, MD, 1995. American Hospital Formulary Service. American Society of Health-System Pharmacists. (800-657-4348)

Case Studies Workbook. Ed: Lem K. Washington, DC, 1993. American Pharmaceutical Association.

Drug Evaluations Annual 1995. Chicago, IL. Divison of Drugs and Toxicology. American Medical Association. (800-621-8335)

Drug Evaluations Subscription. Chicago, IL. American Medical Association. (quarterly plus newsletter) (800-621-8335)

Drug Facts and Comparisons. St. Louis, MO. Facts and Comparisons, Annually. (800-223-0554)

Handbook of Nonprescription Drugs. 10th ed. Washington, DC, 1993. American Pharmaceutical Association. (800-237-2742)

Armstrong L, Lipsy R, Lance L. Drug Information Handbook, 2nd Ed. Washington, D.C. 1994-95. American Pharmaceutical Association. (800-237-2742)

Medication Teaching Manual: A Guide for Patient Counseling. 6th ed. Bethesda, MD, 1995. American Society of Health-System Pharmacists. (301-657-4348)

Patient Counseling Handbook. Washington, DC, 1985. American Pharmaceutical Association. (800-237-2742)

Smith DL. Medication Guide for Patient Counseling. Philadelphia, 1981. Lea & Febiger.

USP DI. Volume I: Drug Information for the Health Care Professional; Volume II: Advice for the Patient. Rockville, MD, 1995. The United States Pharmacopoeial Convention. (800-227-8772)

Computer Resources

AskRx™ Plus, Camdat Corporation, San Bruno, CA. (800-771-7448)

CCIS—The Computerized Clinical Information System, Micromedex, Englewood, DO. (800-525-9083)

Electronic Drug Reference. Englewood, CO: Clinical Reference Systems, Ltd. (800-237-8401)

Maven™, Synthesys Technologies, Inc., Austin, Texas. (800-695-9857)

MedScreen II DDB. Sylmar, CA: MedScreen, Inc. (818-362-5511)

STAT!-Ref™ CD ROM Medical Reference Libraries. Teton Data Systems, Jackson, WY. (800-755-STAT)

USP DI. Volume I: Drug Information for the Health Care Professional; Volume II: Advice for the Patient. Rockville, MD, 1995. The United States Pharmacopoeial Convention. (800-227-8772)

Resources for Patient Counseling and Communication Skills
Print Resources

Bernstein L, Bernstein R. Interviewing: A Guide for Health Professionals. New York, 1990. Appleton-Century-Crofts.

Carnegie D. How to Develop Self-Confidence and Influence People by Public Speaking. New York, 1956. Pocket Book 5 (a division of Simon and Schuster, Inc.).

Communicating the Benefits and Risks of Prescription Drugs (Monograph No. 106) Washington, DC: Center for Risk Communication, Columbia University, School of Public Health. (202-338-2156)

Davis H, Fallowfield L, Ed. Counselling and Communication in Health Care. Chichester, England, 1991. John Wiley & Sons.

Directory of Prescription Medicine Information and Education Programs and Resources and Services. Washington, DC. annually. National Council on Patient Information and Education (NCPIE) (202-347-6711)

Elder J. Transactional Analysis in Health Care. Menlo Park, CA, 1978. Addison-Wesley Publishing Company.

Gerard BA, Boniface W, Love B. Interpersonal Skills for Health Professionals. Reston, VA, 1980. Reston Publishing.

Gundin W, Mammen E. The Art of Speaking Made Simple. Rev. ed. Garden City, NY, 1981. Doubleday and Co.

Hussar D. The Pharmacist's Role in Understanding and Improving Patient Compliance. Alexandria, VA, 1993. (NARD) (800-544-7447)

Klein-Schwartz, W, Hoopes, J. Patient Assessment and Consultation. In: Handbook of Nonprescription Drugs. 10th ed. Washington, DC, 1993. American Pharmaceutical Association.

Knapp ML. Nonverbal Communication in Human Interaction. New York, 1978. Holt, Rinehart & Winston.

Morris L. Communicating Therapeutic Risks. New York, NY, 1990. Springer-Verlag, New York, Inc.

Myerscough P. Talking with Patients—A Basic Clinical Skill. 2nd ed. Oxford, England, 1992. Oxford University Press.

NCPIE NEWS. Washington, DC. quarterly. National Council on Patient Information and Education (NCPIE) (202-347-6711)

The One Minute Counselor. In: American Pharmacy, monthly issues.

Rogers CB. On Becoming a Person. Boston, MA., 1961. Houghton-Mifflin.

Russell C, Wilcox E, Hicks C. Interpersonal Communication in Pharmacy: An Interactionist Approach. New York, 1982. Appleton-Century-Crofts.

Smith DL. Patient and His Medications. In: Medication Guide for Patient Counseling. Philadelphia, 1981. Lea & Febiger.

Smith M. When I Say No, I Feel Guilty. New York, 1975. Dial Press.

Stanaszek W, et al. Understanding Medical Terms: A Guide for Pharmacy Lancaster, PA, 1992. Practice. Technomic Pub. Co.

Steptoe A, Mathews A. Health Care and Human Behaviour. London, England, 1984. Academic Press.

Successful Pharmacy Communication Ideas That Work. NARD/Marion Merrell Dow. Kansas City, MO, 1992. Marion Merrell Dow, Inc., Pharmacy Relations.

Talk About Prescriptions. Month planning guide. Washington, DC. annually. National Council on Patient Information and Education (NCPIE) (202-347-6711)

Tindall W, Beardsley R, Kimberlin C. Communication Skills in Pharmacy Practice: A Practical Guide for Students and Practitioners. 3rd ed. Philadelphia, 1996. Lea & Febiger.

Pharmacists Training Programs

Barnard D, Barr J, Schumacher G. Empathy. Person to Person: The AACP-Lilly Pharmacy Communication Skills Project. Bethesda, MD, 1985. American Association of Colleges of Pharmacy. (Booklet and Videotape)

Barnard D, Barr J, Schumacher G. Nonverbal Communication. Person to Person: The AACP-Lilly Pharmacy Communication Skills Project. Bethesda, MD, 1985. American Association of Colleges of Pharmacy. (Booklet and Videotape)

Counseling Low-Literate Patients. Chapel Hill, NC: North Carolina Pharmaceutical Association. (Videotape and Guide) (800-852-7343)

Gardner M, Boyce R, Herrier R Counseling to Enhance Compliance. Rockville, MD, 1995. U.S. Public Health Service, Indian Health Service/Roerig Division of Pfizer Pharmaceuticals. (Booklet and Videotape) (212-573-7877)

Gardner M, Boyce R, Herrier R. How to Counsel Patients in Challenging Situations. Rockville, MD, 1995. U.S. Public Health Service, Indian Health Service/Roerig Division of Pfizer Pharmaceuticals. (Booklet and Videotape) (212-573-7877)

Gardner M, Boyce R, Herrier R. Pharmacist-Patient Consultation Program. An Interactive Approach to Verify Patient Understanding. Rockville, MD, 1991. U.S. Public Health Service, Indian Health Service/Roerig Division of Pfizer Pharmaceuticals. (Booklet and Videotape) (212-573-7877)

Health Literacy Project. Philadelphia, PA: Health Promotion Council of S.E. Pennsylvania, Inc. (Videotape) (215-546-1276)

Kimberlin C, Lemberger M, Maple Ml Self-Assurance in Pharmacy Practice. Person to Person: The AACP-Lilly Pharmacy Communication Skills Project. Bethesda, MD: American Association of Colleges of Pharmacy. (Booklet and Videotape)

Love D, Wiese. Pharmacy Communication Skills. Chapel Hill, NC, 1982. Health Sciences Consortium. (Videotape)

McKenzie M, Johnson S, Maple M, et al. The Medication History Interview. Chapel Hill, NC, 1981. Health Sciences Consortium. (Booklet and Videotape)

PharmWrite, Improving Pharmacist-Patient Communications. U.S. Pharmacopeial Convention Inc. and Marion Merrel Dow Inc. 1994. (800-227-8772)

Strategies for Better Communication for a Multicultural and Ethnically Diverse Patient Population. OBRA'90: Legislative Overview and Patient Counseling Skills Workshop. U.S. Pharmacopeial Convention Inc. (800-227-8772)

Sumner E, Durand R. Problems in Geriatric Pharmacy. Chapel Hill, NC, 1985. Health Sciences Consortium. (Videotape and Guide)

Resources for Patients to Use
Information for Patients about Medications
Books and Booklets

AARP Pharmacy Service Prescription Drug Handbook. 2nd ed. Alexandria, VA: AARP Pharmacy Service. (800-456-2277)

About Your Medicines. 7th ed. Washington, DC, 1995. U.S. Pharmacopeial Convention, Inc.(800-227-8772)

The AMA Guide to Prescription and Over-the-Counter Drugs. New York, NY, 1988. Random House. (800-733-3000)

The Complete Drug Reference. Des Moines, IA, 1995. Consumer Report Books. (800-272-0722)

Consumers Guide to Prescription Medicines. Washington, DC: Pharmaceutical Manufacturers Association.(202-835-3450)

For Seniors Only: A Guide to Using Drugs in the Later Years. San Francisco, CA: SRx: Medication Education for Seniors, San Francisco Department of Public Health. (415-554-3274)

Hodgson Brown E, Paige Walker L. The Informed Consumer's Pharmacy. The Essential Guide to Prescription and Over-the-Counter Drugs. NY, 1990. Carroll & Graf Publisher Inc.

Guidebooks to Medicine Series (Pediatrics, Senior Adult, Arthritis, Diabetes, Women's, and Men's & Sports Medicine). Atlanta, GA: Federal Medical Reports, Inc. (404-993-9692)

Long, James. The essential guide to prescription drugs. NY, 1991. Harper Collins.

Over-the-Counter Medications: A Guide for Older Adults. San Francisco, CA: SRx: Medication Education for Seniors, San Francisco Department of Public Health. (415-554-3274)

USP. Drug Information for the Consumer. Mount Vernon, NY, 1990. Consumers Union.(800-227-8772)

USP DI: Volume II—Advice for the Patient. Washington, DC, 1995. U.S. Pharmacopeial Convention, Inc. (800-227-8772)

Leaflets

AMA Patient Medication Instructions. Rockville, MD: U.S. Pharmacopeial Convention Inc. (800-227-8772)

CMA Guide to Prescription and Over-the-Counter Drugs. Ottawa, Canada, 1990. Canadian Medical Association. (613-731-9331)

Drug Information Card Sets. Chapel Hill, NC: UNC Hospitals. (919-966-1091)

Medication Information Leaflets for Seniors. Alexandria, VA: AARP Pharmacy Service. (703-684-0244)

Medication Fact Sheets. San Francisco, CA: SRx: Medication Education for Seniors. (415-544-3274)

Pamphlets from Pharmaceutical manufacturers—for a list of available materials see: Sources: A Catalog of Information Materials on Medicine and Health Available from the Pharmaceutical Industry. Washington, DC: Pharmaceutical Manufacturers Association. (202-835-3450)

Pamphlets from National Council on Patient Information and Education (NCPIE). Washington, DC. (202-347-6711)

Patient Advisory Leaflets. New Smyrna Beach, FL: ABP/PHARMEX.

Patient Drug Facts. St. Louis, MO: Facts and Comparisons. (800-223-0554)

Patient Information Leaflets. Alexandria, VA: National Association of Retail Druggists. (NARD) (800-544-7447)

Patient Medication Instruction Sheets. Elk Grove Village, IL: American Academy of Pediatrics. (708-228-5005)

Smith DL. Family Guide to Canadian Prescription Drugs. Unionville, Canada, 1986. Pharmasystems, Inc. (905-475-2500)

Smith DL. Family Guide to Prescription Drugs, Willimantic, CN, 1982. ABP/PHARMEX. (800-233-0585)

Smith DL. Patient Guide to Prescription Drugs, Willimantic, CN, 1982. ABP/PHARMEX. (800-233-0585)

Smith DL. Understanding Prescription Drugs. New York, NY, 1989. Simon & Schuster.

Smith DL. Understanding Canadian Prescription Drugs. Toronto, Canada, 1992. Key Porter Books.

Some Facts About Giving Liquid Medicine to Your Infant; Some Facts About Giving Liquid Medicine to Your Toddler; Some Facts About Giving Capsules, Pills or Tablets to Your Child. Chapel Hill, NC: UNC Hospitals. (919-966-1091)

USP DI Patient Education Leaflet Products. Rockville, MD: U.S. Pharmacopeial Convention Inc. (800-227-8772)

Computerized Information

Healthtouch. Cambridge, MA: Medical Strategies. (800-825-3742)

Mayo Clinic Family Pharmacist. Eden Prairie, MN: IVI Publishing. (800-754-1484)

Medication Advisor. Englewood, CO: Clinical Reference Systems, Ltd. (800-237-8401)

Medication Advisory Center. New Smyrna Beach, FL: ABP/PHARMEX. (800-233-0585)

MedScreen II DDB. Sylmar, CA: MedScreen, Inc. (818-362-5511)

Medteach. Bethesda, MD. American Society of Health-System Pharmacists. (301-657-4348)

Patient Drug Education Database™. Indianapolis, IN: Medi-Span, Inc. (800-428-4495)

RxTriage. San Bruno, CA: First DataBank-The Hearst Corp. (800-633-3453)

The USP DI Patient Education Leaflet™ Database. Rockville, MD: The United States Pharmacopeial Convention, Inc. (800-227-8772)

USP DI Volume II, Advice for the Patient Database.Rockville, MD, 1995. The United States Pharmacopeial Convention, Inc. (800-227-8772)

Information about Medical Problems in General or Specific Conditions

Pamphlets and Videotape Materials

Adult Health Advisor. Englewood, CO: Clinical Reference Systems Ltd. (800-237-8401)

Go Ahead, Ask Your Pharmacist. Bethesda, MD: American Society of Health-System Pharmacists. (301-657-4348)

Health Literacy Project-Patient Materials. Philadelphia, PA: Health Promotion Council of S.E. Pennsylvania, Inc. (215-546-1276)

MedScreen. (interactive diagnostic software program) Sylmar, CA: MedScreen, Inc. (818-362-5511)

The Personal Health Center (interactive video). Columbus, OH: Advanced Interactive Video, Inc. (614-291-2777)

Take Charge! True Stories of Patients Who Won. Roswell, FA: Florida Health Care Information Council. (404-640-9240)

Understanding Your Prescription; How to Manage Your Medication; Prescription Medications for Mental Health; Why Adults Need Shots. Rockville, MD: U.S. Pharmacopeial Convention. (800-227-8772)

USP Visualized: About Your Diabetes (interactive video). Rockville, MD: U.S. Pharmacopeial Convention. (800-227-8772)

Many organizations provide a variety of pamphlets and some videotapes designed for patients. Most of these organizations have local, state, or national offices. Contact the local branch for a list of available pamphlets. The following is by no means a complete list of these organizations:

Alzheimer's Association
American Cancer Society
American Diabetes Association
American Lung Association
American Liver Foundation
American Association of Retired Persons
Arthritis Foundation
Asthma and Allergy Foundation of America
Council on Family Health
Epilepsy Foundation
Lupus Foundation of America
March of Dimes Birth Defects Foundation
Medic Alert Foundation International
National Association for Sickle Cell Disease
National Society to Prevent Blindness
National Osteoporosis Foundation
National Mental Health Association
National Kidney Foundation
National Consumers League
National Council on Aging
National Council on Patient Information and Education
Spina Bifida Association of America

Various government departments also provide information pamphlets for patients on a variety of topics:

Office of Disease Prevention and Health Promotion, National Health Information Center, Washington, DC.
FDA/Office of Consumer Affairs, Consumer Inquiries Section, Rockville, MD.

Pharmaceutical manufacturers—individual companies and associations (pamphlets and videotaped materials):

Nonprescription Drug Manufacturers Association, Washington, DC.
Pharmaceutical Manufacturers Association, Washington, DC.

Planned Programs for Pharmacists to Use In Educating Patients

Brown Bag Medicine Revue Starter Kit. Washington, DC. National Council on Patient Information and Education (NCPIE) (202-347-6711)

Brown Bag Prescription Evaluation Clinic Manual. 3rd ed. Kingston, RI:College of Pharmacy, University of Rhode Island. (401-792-2789)

Other assistance with planning a brown bag program available from: California Pharmacists Association, Sacramento, CA. (800-444-3851)

Elder-Health Program. Baltimore, MD: University of Maryland, School of Pharmacy. (301-328-3243)

Go Ahead, Ask Your Pharmacist. Bethesda, MD: American Society of Health-System Pharmacists. (800-657-4348)

Katy's Kids Education Kit. Des Moines, IA: Iowa Pharmacy Foundation. (515-270-0713)

Managing Your Medicines As You Grow Older. Washington, DC: American Pharmaceutical Association.(800-237-2742)

Medication Education Mini-Class Curriculum Guides. San Francisco, CA: SRx: Medication Education for Seniors. (415-554-3274)

Medicine is No Mystery. 5087 Washington, DC 20061-5087: National Council on the Aging. Publication Dept.

National Medication Awareness Test. Washington, DC: American Pharmaceutical Association. (800-237-2742)

The Other Drug Problem: Medication Misuse Among Older Americans. Project Pride, Rockville, MD. (videotape) (301-251-9639)

Prescription Patrol. Manitowoc, WI: Newsworthy Ink. (414-682-8191)

Self Medication Awareness Test. Washington, DC: American Pharmaceutical Association. (800-237-2742)

What You Don't Know About Drugs Can Hurt You. Alexandria, VA: National Association Retail Druggists. (800-544-7447)

Adapted from : NCPIE. Talk About Prescriptions Month. Planning Guide. Washington, DC: National Council on Patient Information and Education. October, 1992.

Author's Note: Inclusion in this list does not indicate evaluation or endorsement of the product. Pharmacists must make their own evaluations as recommended in Chapter 6.

APPENDIX B

SUGGESTED PATIENT-COUNSELING DIALOGUES

The following dialogues are provided to assist pharmacists in the patient-counseling discussion, in particular, ways to introduce topics, and ways to word difficult concepts like side effects. Of course this is just a suggestion, and the pharmacist should use words with which he or she feels natural and comfortable. Please note also that, since this does not include patient dialogue, real-life counseling may result in a slightly different organization as discussed in Chapter 8.

Counseling for a New Prescription
Opening Discussion

a. Personal introduction:

> *"Hello, Mrs. Jones. I'm the pharmacist, Melanie."*

b. Exchange pleasantries where appropriate:

> *"Nice weather we're having today?"*

c. Explain the purpose of the counseling session:

> *"I'd just like to take a few minutes to discuss your prescription with you to make sure you get the most benefit from it."*

d. Give written information if available:

> *"Here is some information about your medication. Read it over when you get home, and if you have any questions, give us a call."*

Discussion to Gather Information and Identify Problems

a. Medication history:

- If the patient is new to the pharmacy, conduct a medication-history interview. See the dialogue in the Medication-History Interview section.

- If the patient is already on record, confirm before embarking on counseling that he has not had this medication before and that the situation therefore requires new-prescription counseling.

b. Patient's present knowledge:

- Find out what the patient knows about the medication and the reason that he or she must take it:

> *"What did the doctor tell you about the medication?"*

- If necessary, also ask:

> *"How did the doctor say it would help?"*

> *"What did he/she say it was for?"*

c. Potential problems

- Identify potential problems. Ask:

    "Do you have any questions or concerns about anything at this point."

- Discuss problems identified when preparing the prescription. Say:

    "I have a concern about..."

    "I need to ask you more about..."

- Summarize problems identified and rank. Say:

    "It seems we have a few things to discuss. First I think we need to..."

Discussion to Prevent or Resolve Problems and Give Information

a. Discuss problems ranked as needed.

b. Proceed to provide information as needed:

(i)   What the medication is called:

   "This medication is called _____."

(ii)   What the medication is supposed to do (if the patient doesn't know):

   "They are pain killers, to relieve the pain in your back."

(iii) How and when to take the medication:

   "How did the doctor tell you to take it?"

   If the patient doesn't know, tell them, for example:

   "Take them every 3 to 4 hours, but only when you need them for the pain. It's best to take them with food or milk so that the aspirin won't upset your stomach."

(iv)   Compliance discussion:

   "Do you see any difficulties in taking this as I've suggested?"

   If suggestions seem necessary:

   "You may find it easier to remember to take the pills if you always take them at meal times."

(v)   Precautions or side effects:

   "Sometimes along with the wanted effect of the drug, unexpected effects occur. Did the doctor mention anything about this?"

   - Mention only the most common side effects and only those that are appropriate (e.g., warn against sun exposure only in summer or if the patient spends prolonged periods out of doors).

- Include instructions on how to minimize or avoid side effects:

   "Some people find that these pills make them drowsy, so see how they affect you before you drive or do anything that requires alertness."

(vi) Symptoms of adverse effects:

   - Mention only the most common adverse effects, and put them into perspective by noting how rarely they occur. Describe the signs of adverse effects (do not give complicated names) and what to do if they arise:

   "Very rarely (occasionally, frequently), people develop a reaction to this medication. This probably won't happen to you, but if you notice an unexplained fever or a rash, let your doctor or the pharmacist know about it right away."

(vii) Storage instructions, if any.

(viii) Refill instructions:

   "The doctor has written that you may get these pills again in 10 days if you still need them."

   - If there are no refill instructions and it's a medication that would likely be refilled, find out if the doctor instructed the patient verbally:

   "Did the doctor tell you what to do when you finish these pills?"

c. Discuss outcomes and monitoring:

   "You should be feeling some relief of pain within 30 minutes of taking this medication. Let me or your doctor know if you are not finding relief. Hopefully by the time you have finished all these pills, you'll no longer be needing it."

Closing Discussion

a. Recap important points:

   "Remember, this medication may make you drowsy."

b. Get feedback:

   - Make sure the patient understands:

   "Do you have any questions about this?"

   - If the directions are complicated or if you doubt that the patient has understood them, ask the patient to repeat the directions back to you:

   "Just to make sure I've made myself clear, could you tell me now how you are going to take these pills?"

c. Encourage the patient to call if any questions or problems arise:

> *"If you have any questions or problems, don't hesitate to call us."*

d. Arrange follow-up:

> *"Would you give me a call towmorrow to let me know how you are doing with the medication?"*

> • Alternatively: *"Can I call you tomorrow to see how you are doing with the medication?...What time would be convenient?"*

Follow-Up Discussions

a. Introduce yourself as above.

b. Remind the patient why you are calling:

> *"I'm calling to make sure you're getting the desired effect from the medication."*

c. Follow with specific questions:

> *"Are you finding it helps the symptom or condition being treated?"*

> *"Are you finding any difficulty taking it?"*

> *"How often are you taking it?"*

> *"How do you feel when you take it?"*

> *"Have you noticed any upset stomach at all?"*

d. Provide suggestions or advice where appropriate.

e. Close as for the main counseling discussion.

Refill Prescription Counseling and Medication Monitoring

Opening Discussion

a. Personal introduction (including both the patient's name and your name if you're not already acquainted):

> *"Hello, Mrs. Jones. I'm the pharmacist, _____."*

b. Exchange pleasantries where appropriate:

> *"Nice weather we're having today?"*

c. Explain the purpose of the counseling session:

> *"I'd just like to discuss your prescription with you for a few minutes to make sure you're getting the most benefit from it."*

Discussion to Gather Information and Identify Problems

a. Medication history:

- Check the patient record before counseling for any new medications that could cause problems in combination with this one (e.g., scheduling, drug interactions). To confirm that there are no changes ask the patient:

  "Are you on any new medications that were prescribed by a doctor or that you purchased yourself, since you were last here?"

b. General inquiry:

- Ask the patient if he or she has any questions about or has had any problems with taking the medication:

  "Is there anything you'd like to discuss about this medication?"

e. Effectiveness:

- Ask the patient if the medication is having the desired effect:

  "Are you finding it helps the symptom or condition being treated?"

d. Compliance:

- Ask the patient if he or she has any problems with taking the medication:

  "Are you finding any difficulty taking it?"

- Determine whether the patient is compliant by checking the date of the last refill and by asking how he or she takes the medication:

  "When during the day do you take the pills?"

- If you suspect noncompliance, probe further, without sounding judgmental:

  "It's sometimes difficult to find the time to take your medication. How often would you say you miss a dose?"

e. Side effects or adverse effects:

- Find out if the patient is experiencing any untoward effects:

  "Have you noticed anything unusual or out of the ordinary while taking this?"

- Be more specific, if necessary, naming possible symptoms of adverse effects or side effects:

  "Have you had an upset stomach at all while you've been taking this?"

Discussion to Prevent or Resolve Problems and Give Information

Give information about the illness and the drug where necessary regarding any compliance or side-effect problems detected or other questions or problems mentioned by the patient, for example:

> *"You might find this medication less irritating to your stomach if you take it at meal times or with some food or milk"*

or

> *"This medication is not intended to actually cure your back problems. It will just help to relieve the pain."*

or

> *"This medication may be more effective if you take it on a regular basis when your back is bothering you a lot, rather than waiting until the pain is extreme."*

Closing Discussion

Same as for new prescription.

a. Recap important points or provide reassurance as needed;

b. Get feedback;

c. Encourage the patient to call if any questions or problems arise;

d. Arrange follow-up.

Follow-up Discussion

As discussed above for new prescription counseling.

Nonprescription Drug Counseling

Opening Discussion

a. Personal introduction:

> *"I'm the pharmacist, _____. Can I help you find something?"*

b. Find out for whom the over-the-counter drug is intended:

> *"Who is the medication for?"*

c. Explain the purpose of the counseling session:

> *"I'll just ask you a few questions to find out the best medication for you in this situation."*

d. Provide print information, if available:

>   *"Here is some information about colds."*

Discussion to Gather Information and Identify Problems

a. If the patient is not present, find out his or her age.

b. Medication history and chronic conditions:

>   - If you have a patient record for this patient, check it before counseling to see whether the patient is currently taking any medications or has any conditions that might interfere with nonprescription medication use.
>
>   - If the patient is new, conduct a brief medication history:
>
>   *"I need to ask you a few questions about your health."*
>
>   *"Are you taking any other medications at the moment?"*
>
>   *"Have you ever had a reaction to any drug that you've taken before?"*
>
>   *"Do you have any medical conditions at the moment, such as diabetes, high blood pressure, heart condition, ulcer, and so on?"*

c. Patient's present situation:

>   - Find out if the patient has consulted a doctor or a pharmacist about this condition before:
>
>   *"Have you spoken to your doctor or a pharmacist about this before?...What did he tell you to do?"*

d. History of condition:

>   *"How long have you had this?"*
>
>   *"Have you ever had it before?"*

e. Description of symptoms:

>   *"Is the cough dry and tickly? ... Is it loose and rattley?"*

f. Past treatment:

>   *"What have you taken already or in the past for this condition? ... How well did it work?"*

Discussion to Prevent or Resolve Problems and Give Information

a. If no medication is warranted or if it appears necessary to see the doctor, then recommend this:

> *"It seems that the best thing for you would be to continue using the humidifier and the medication the doctor gave you already."*

or

> *"In your case, I think it's best not to take anything right now. I suggest you see your doctor as soon as possible."*

b. Recommendation:

- Give information about the condition. Suggest nondrug remedies if possible. If appropriate, suggest a product to use. Be supportive and encouraging:

  > *"Your cough sounds like it's a tickly cough resulting from your cold and runny nose. It will probably improve as the cold gets better."*

  > *"Try having frequent sips of juice or water, and try sucking cough candies to ease the tickle."*

  > *"This cough medicine may help dry up your runny nose and reduce your coughing."*

c. Product information:

- If a product is recommended, give information about the medication as described for prescription counseling: name, purpose, directions, side effects, and precautions, etc.

Closing Discussion

a. Recap important points.

b. Get feedback:

- Make sure the patient understands:

  > *"Do you have any questions about this?"*

c. Whether a medication is recommended or not, suggest that the patient contact his or her physician if the condition persists:

> *"If this continues on for _____ days, or seems to get worse _____ (give specific signs if appropriate, e.g., green sputum), then see your doctor."*

d. If the directions are complicated or if you doubt that the patient has understood them, ask him or her to repeat the directions:

"Just to make sure I've made myself clear, could you tell me now how you are going to take this cough medicine?"

e. Encourage to call if any questions or problems arise:

"If you have any questions or problems, don't hesitate to call us."

d. Arrange follow-up: Same as for new prescription.

Follow-up Discussion

Same as for new prescription counseling.

Medication-History Interview
Opening Discussion

a. Personal introduction:

"Hello, Mrs. Jones. I'm the pharmacist, _____."

b. Exchanging pleasantries where appropriate:

"Nice weather we're having today?"

c. Explain the purpose of the medication-history interview:

"In this pharmacy, we keep records about you and the medications you take to help ensure that you get the most benefit from them. I'd like to take a few minutes to ask you some questions."

d. Ensure confidentiality:

"Of course, any information you give me will be strictly confidential and will be kept in the computer in your personal patient record."

e. Get consent:

"Would it be all right for me to continue with this now?"

or

"I'd like to continue with this now."

Inquiry of Personal Information

a. Introduce the section:

"First I need some information for our records about yourself."

b. Ask personal questions:

"Sometime your age or what you do for a living can affect your health and medication use so I need to ask you about these."

"What is your birth date?"

"Are you working at the moment?...Do you mind telling me what you do?"

Some comments following the patient's responses would help set a conversational tone, e.g., *"That's the same month as my birthday...That sounds like an interesting job."*

c. Use of health-care professionals

"Who is your family doctor?...How often do you see him/her?"

"Do you also see any specialists?...What is your dermatologist's name?...How often do you see him/her?"

Discussion of Medical Conditions and Medication Use

a. Introduce the section:

"Now I'd like to ask about your medical conditions and medication use."

b. Ask about the condition currently being treated:

"First, what brought you to the doctor?"

c. About existing conditions in general:

"Do you have any medical conditions at the moment, such as diabetes, high blood pressure, heart condition, ulcer, and so on?"

d. Gather information about each condition and the medications associated with it before proceeding to the next condition.

- Ask about the duration of the condition:

"Now I'd like to discuss each of your conditions. First, how long have you had diabetes?"

- Ask about medication used for the condition:

"Are you taking any medication at the moment for your diabetes?"

- Ask details about each medication sequentially:

1. Prescriber: *"Who prescribed this medication for you?"*

2. Method of use: *"How do you take this medication?"*

- Probe for details, if necessary, to ascertain compliance:

"How much do you take each time?"

"When during the day do you take it?"

"When do you take it in relation to meal times?"

"How many days a week do you take it, on average?"

3. Effectiveness: *"Do you find that these pills help you?"*

4. Reasons for noncompliance (if noncompliance is detected):

"Is there any particular reason that you don't take this every day?"

or

"I realize it's difficult to remember to take medications on a regular basis. Is that a problem for you?"

5. Side effects and adverse effects:

"Have you noticed anything unusual or out of the ordinary while taking this?"

- Be more specific, if necessary, naming possible symptoms of adverse effects or side effects:

"Have you had an upset stomach at all while you've been taking this?"

e. Repeat (1–5) for each medication.

f. Past medications for the condition:

"Have you been on any other medications for this condition in the past?"

"Why were they discontinued?"

g. Repeat (c–e) for each condition.

h. Other prescribed medication use:

"Other than the medications we've discussed, are there any other medications that you take?"

Nonprescription Drug Use

a. Names of nonprescription drugs used:

"Are there any medications that you take that you buy yourself without a prescription?

"Do you take any herbal or home remedies?"

- Probe if necessary:

"Do you take anything for stomach upset?...What about for colds?...for headaches or pain?"

b. Method of use:

   1. Dosage:

      "How much do you take each time?"

   2. Frequency:

      "When do you take it during the day?"

   3. Duration:

      "Are you taking this at present?"

      "How often do you take this. . .most days?

      "How often have you used this in the past few weeks?

   4. Side effects or adverse effects:

- Find out if the patient is experiencing any untoward effects:

  "Have you noticed anything unusual or out of the ordinary while taking this?"

- Be more specific, if necessary, naming only possible symptoms of adverse effects or side effects:

  "Have you had an upset stomach at all while you've been taking this?"

Discussion of Alcohol and Tobacco Use

a. Introduce the topic:

      "Now, I need to ask you about alcohol and tobacco use. This is important for me to know since alcohol and tobacco can affect your conditions and your medications."

b. Proceed with a question about smoking:

      "Do you smoke at all?"

c. Ask about alcohol use:

      "Most people have a glass of wine or beer with their meals or in the evenings. How often would you have an alcoholic beverage?...Do you alter the way you take your medication when you are planning to have a drink?"

Discussion of Allergies or Drug Sensitivities

a. Ask about allergies:

> *"Are you allergic to any medication that you know of?"*

b. If the answer is yes, ask the patient to describe the reaction:

> *"What happened when you took _____?"*

c. Ask if the present physician is aware of this:

> *"Does Dr. _____ know about this?"*

d. Ask about any previous problems with drug use:

> *"Have you ever had an unpleasant or untoward effect from a medication?"*

e. If the answer is yes, repeat (b) and (c).

Closing Discussion

a. Ask if there is any other information the patient thinks you should know:

> *"We're just about finished now. Is there any other information you think I should know?"*

b. Tell the patient what will be done with the information and whether you will need to consult with him or her further:

> *"I'll be keeping this information on your medication record for future reference."*

or

> *"There are a few more things that I'd like to discuss with you about your medications. Could we meet again [arrange a time if possible] ?"*

or

> *"I'll be looking this over and will probably meet with you again when you are discharged from hospital."*

c. Thank the patient for his or her time:

> *"Thank you for your time and help."*

Assessment and Documentation

a. Introduction:

- Introduce yourself as above

- Introduce the discussion

  "When we talked...(earlier, yesterday, last week, etc.)...I asked you quite a few questions about your health and medication use. I've thought it over and there's a few things I'd like to discuss with you that might help you to get more benefit from your medications."

b. Proceed to discuss issues and make recommendations as necessary.

APPENDIX C

FORMS TO ASSIST IN INFORMATION GATHERING

Medication-History Interview Form

When conducting a patient-history interview, it is helpful for the pharmacist to use a medication-history interview form to gather data. This form can also be used to document the history-taking activity and to note any interventions that the pharmacist decides to make as follow-up to the interview.

Patient Questionnaire

In order to save time conducting a medication-history interview, a patient questionnaire can be used. The pharmacist should explain the purpose of the medication history interview then ask the patient to complete the form while they wait for their prescription to be prepared. When it is complete, the pharmacist can then review the information on it with the patient, asking questions where more detailed information is needed.

Nonprescription Drug Counseling Recording Form

When counseling patients regarding nonprescription drugs, it is useful to have a form to record information gathered during the discussion with the patient. It can also serve as documentation of the counseling encounter for the pharmacist's records and, if necessary, to send to the patient's physician.

One part of the form listing the pharmacist's suggestions for treatment can also be separated and given to the patient for their future reference.

MEDICATION HISTORY INTERVIEW FORM

Patient Name:_____ **Date:**_____
Birth Date:_____ **Drug Plan:**_____
Physicians: _____

1. Conditions *(duration):* Primary concern today:_____
  Kidney disease _____   Heart Disease _____   Diabetes _____
  Liver disease _____   High blood pressure _____   Thyroid disease _____
  Stomach or   Asthma, Bronchitis ____   Epsilepsy _____
   duodenal ulcer _____   Hay fever or
  Other: _____   other allergies _____

2. Medications currently used for each condition:
Condition #1

Drug Name	Dose	Freq/day	Duration	Effectiveness	ADR

Condition #2

Drug Name	Dose	Freq/day	Duration	Effectiveness	ADR

Condition #3

Drug Name	Dose	Freq/day	Duration	Effectiveness	ADR

3. Over-the-counter/Herbal/Homeopathic/Home Remedies

Drug Name	Dose	Freq/day	Duration	Effectiveness	ADR

4. Adverse Effects:

Drug	Effects

5. Drug-related Problems and Recommendations:

Problem	Alternatives	Recommendation

6. Interventions:
Patient counseled:_____   Physician contacted: _____
Other:

PATIENT QUESTIONNAIRE

NAME: _____   _____

Note: All information given in this questionnaire will be kept strictly confidential.

This pharmacy keeps records about you and the medication you take to help ensure that you get the most benefit from your medication. The pharmacist may want to spend a few minutes with you to discuss the use of your medication in confidence, and at no cost to you, when your prescription is ready. To allow the pharmacist to accurately assess your medications, please answer the following questions:

1. Do you have any chronic illnesses? *(If yes, please check below)*

                                    ✍ yes   ✍ no

• Kidney disease	• Heart disease	• Diabetes
• Liver disease	• High blood pressure	• Thyroid disease
• Stomach or	• Asthma, Bronchitis	• Epilepsy
duodenal ulcer	• Hay fever or other allergies	
• Other:	_____	

2. What medications are you currently taking on a regular basis? How much are you taking per day?

Prescription drugs	Dose	Freq/day	Physician

Over-the-Counter, Herbal, or Home Remedies:

	Purpose	Dose	Freq/day
Laxative			
Headache pills			
Antacids			
Cold & allergy remedies			

3. Have you ever experienced any ill effects from medications? yes__ no__
   If yes, please describe:

Drug	Ill effects

Thank you.

NONPRESCRIPTION COUNSELING RECORDING FORM

Date: _____

Patient Name: _____ Age: _____

Address: _____ Phone: _____

Medication History

Illness Conditions:–See patient record____ or Form attached____

Physician's Name:_____ Consulted: Yes___   No___

Presenting Complaint

Location:_____

Quality:_____

Severity:_____

Modifying factors:_____

Timing:_____

Associated symptoms:_____

Previous treatment:_____

Recommended time for follow-up:_____

Copy and tear here for the patient

....

Pharmacist's Suggestions for Treatment

Patient's name:_____

Contact physician:_____

Nonmedication recommendations:_____

Nonprescription medication:_____

Information provided (As per label):_____

Additional information:_____

If the condition worsens or does not improve within_____
contact the pharmacist or your physician.

Pharmacist:_____ Date:_____

Adapted From: Srnka Q. Implementing a self-care-consulting practice. Am Pharm. 1993:NS33(1):61-70.

INDEX

Note: Page numbers in italics indicate figures; Page numbers followed by *t* indicate tables.